FAST FACTS FOR THE
GERONTOLOGY NURSE

Charlotte Eliopoulos, RN, MPH, ND, PhD, has demonstrated a commitment to advancing the competencies of nurses who work with older adults through her teaching, writing, and unique leadership roles since the formal recognition of gerontological nursing as a specialty. She has served in a variety of positions ranging from nursing assistant to director of nursing, and pioneered such roles as clinical specialist in gerontological nursing in the acute medical service of the Johns Hopkins Hospital and state specialist in gerontological nursing for the Maryland Department of Health. Currently she is the Executive Director of the American Association for Long-Term Care Nursing.

Dr. Eliopoulos's professional activities have included serving as president of the American Holistic Nursing Association, an active member of the American Nurses Association Committee to revise Gerontological Nursing Standards, a board member of the Advancing Excellence Campaign, honorary member of the National Association of Directors of Nursing Administration (NADONA), and a leader in the Coalition of Geriatric Nursing Organizations. She serves as an advisor to several university-based projects related to leadership in long-term care and gerontological nursing, and has addressed a variety of health care groups nationally and internationally.

As is demonstrated in *Fast Facts for the Gerontology Nurse*, Dr. Eliopoulos has an ability to translate complex theory and research into user-friendly guidelines for practice. In addition to numerous chapters and articles, she has written over 17 books, including *Gerontological Nursing*, 8th Edition, *Invitation to Holistic Health*, 3rd Edition, *Nursing Administration of Long-Term Care*, 7th Edition, *DON Guide for Excellence in LTC, LPN Guide for Excellence in LTC, Staff Development Handbook for Long-Term Care Facilities*, and *Culture Change Nurse Coordinator Manual*.

Springer Publishing Company, LLC
11 West 42nd Street
New York, NY 10036
www.springerpub.com

Acquisitions Editor: Elizabeth A. Nieginski
Composition: S4Carlisle

ISBN: 978-0-8261-9827-3
e-book ISBN: 978-0-8261-9828-0

13 14 15 16 / 5 4 3 2 1

The author and the publisher of this Work have made every effort to use sources believed to be reliable to provide information that is accurate and compatible with the standards generally accepted at the time of publication. Because medical science is continually advancing, our knowledge base continues to expand. Therefore, as new information becomes available, changes in procedures become necessary. We recommend that the reader always consult current research and specific institutional policies before performing any clinical procedure. The author and publisher shall not be liable for any special, consequential, or exemplary damages resulting, in whole or in part, from the readers' use of, or reliance on, the information contained in this book. The publisher has no responsibility for the persistence or accuracy of URLs for external or third-party Internet websites referred to in this publication and does not guarantee that any content on such websites is, or will remain, accurate or appropriate.

Library of Congress Cataloging-in-Publication Data

Eliopoulos, Charlotte, author.
Fast facts for the gerontology nurse : a nursing care guide in a nutshell / Charlotte Eliopoulos.
    p. cm.—(Fast facts)
  Includes bibliographical references and index.
  ISBN-13: 978-0-8261-9827-3 ISBN-10: 0-8261-9827-9 ISBN-13: 978-0-8261-9828-0 (e-book)
  I. Title. II. Series: Fast facts (Springer Publishing Company)
  [DNLM: 1. Geriatric Nursing. WY 152]
  RC954
  618.97'0231—dc23
                            2013035955

Special discounts on bulk quantities of our books are available to corporations, professional associations, pharmaceutical companies, health care organizations, and other qualifying groups. If you are interested in a custom book, including chapters from more than one of our titles, we can provide that service as well.

For details, please contact:
Special Sales Department, Springer Publishing Company, LLC
11 West 42nd Street, 15thFloor, New York, NY 10036-8002
Phone: 877-687-7476 or 212-431-4370; Fax: 212-941-7842
E-mail: sales@springerpub.com

Printed in the United States of America by Gasch Printing.

FAST FACTS FOR THE GERONTOLOGY NURSE
A Nursing Care Guide in a Nutshell

Charlotte Eliopoulos, RN, MPH, ND, PhD

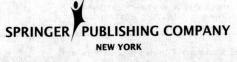

SPRINGER PUBLISHING COMPANY
NEW YORK

Contents

Part III: Special Considerations in Geriatric Care

Preface

Nurses are working with older adults in virtually every care setting and facing the challenges of integrating gerontological nursing knowledge and skills into their practice. Thirteen percent of the
population is over age 65, with growing numbers of baby boomers
adding to it by the day. Of the hospital populations for whom nurses
provide care, 60% are over age 65 and 90% of nursing home residents
are senior adults. Older persons also make up a large percentage of
the population using home health and primary care services. Not
only is the older population presenting in greater numbers, but also
in diversity. In the practice of gerontological nursing, a nurse may:

- Provide postoperative care for a 77 year old who is receiving
  rehabilitation in a subacute care unit following a hip
  replacement
- Counsel a 70-year-old widow who is remarrying and seeking
  advice regarding how to re-establish sexual activity
- Assist a family in safeguarding their home and managing caregiving activities for the 88-year-old relative with dementia
  who is moving in with them
- Educate a group at a local senior citizens' center on health tips
  to avoid cardiovascular disease
- Guide a 65-year-old gay man in finding a lesbian/gay/bisexual/
  transgender (LGBT) support group following the death of his
  partner
- Help a depressed 82 year old who has just been admitted to a
  nursing home carve out a meaningful life

In addition to the unique body of gerontological nursing best practice knowledge, nurses must utilize information from many clinical specialties to competently address the needs of older adults. *Fast Facts for the Gerontology Nurse: A Nursing Care Guide in a Nutshell* offers an efficient means for this to be accomplished. It provides core knowledge that equips nurses to differentiate normal from abnormal findings, understand the unique presentation and management of diseases, and integrate unique age-specific considerations into care planning and implementation with older adults. A holistic approach is used, in which all facets of the individual— physical and mental health, emotional and spiritual well-being, self-care capacity, family relationships and care, unique risks—are addressed. Information is presented in an easy to retrieve style to enable the book to be an effective reference for practice.

The book is divided into three sections:

- Part I, The Older Population and Nursing, lays a basic foundation of the characteristics of the older population and general considerations in applying the nursing process to gerontological care.
- The normal characteristics and major conditions affecting each body system and mental function are presented in Part II, Normalcy and Disease in Late Life. Age-related changes are described, along with guidance on assessing each system and mental status.
- Part III presents Special Considerations in Geriatric Care and offers facts and nursing tips on spirituality, improving functional ability, promoting safety, fostering family health, ensuring safe use of medications, protecting older adults' legal rights, reducing legal risks, and supporting individuals through the dying process. Unique aspects and challenges of caring for older adults in hospitals, nursing homes, home health, and other settings are also reviewed.

The Introduction and Objectives at the beginning of each chapter present an overview of the content that will be presented and what the reader can expect to gain by reading the chapter. Throughout the book the reader will see *Fast Facts in a Nutshell,* which offer information to expand an understanding of the topic discussed and *Clinical*

Snapshots to describe practices that assist with application of content. *Resources* that readers can explore for additional information are listed, as are *Recommended Readings* for those who want to explore additional information on a topic.

For nurses whose primary focus is gerontological care, as well as those for whom geriatric care is a component of another specialty, *Fast Facts for the Gerontology Nurse: A Nursing Care Guide in a Nutshell* should serve as a user-friendly, evidence-based resource that will enhance the quality of care for older adults and foster an understanding of the unique aspects of gerontological nursing.

Charlotte Eliopoulos RN, MPH, ND, PhD

Acknowledgments

It is the rare author who writes a book without the assistance, support, and encouragement of many others. Some of those who contribute to the effort have been actively engaged in specific ways; others have had a more subtle role in impacting the thought and firing the inspiration of the author. These realities cause me to feel cautious and humble as I attempt to acknowledge those who have had a role in this book.

Special appreciation is felt for Elizabeth A. Nieginski, Executive Editor of the Nursing Division at Springer Publishing Company, who had the vision for this book and guided its birth and development. She is truly a gifted professional who is able to provide highly skilled direction while respecting the talent of the author. Her Assistant Editor, Chris Teja, must be acknowledged for attending to the many details behind the scenes that eased my efforts and ensured all loose ends were weaved into an acceptable finished product.

The specialty of gerontological nursing has been rich with nurse leaders who were willing to share and encourage others. I have been fortunate to have benefited from their examples and guidance. Likewise, I have been encouraged by caregivers and older adults who provided insights that aided me in understanding the type of literature that would benefit them the most. They have contributed in more ways than I can begin to identify.

Lastly, I must acknowledge my husband, George Considine, for his patience when the unglamorous aspects of writing caused me to behave in a less than warm and fuzzy manner. His support and optimism mean more than he will ever know.

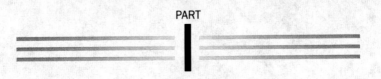

PART

I

The Older Population and Nursing

I

The Older Population

The population aged 65 and over is growing in number and diversity, and creating new challenges for nursing. It can include the 86-year-old nursing home resident with Alzheimer's disease, the 66-year-old widow who wants suggestions on how to have more comfortable sexual relations now that she has found a new partner, the 70-year-old executive with macular degeneration who needs a special device to read a computer screen, and a variety of other profiles. Advances in health care have enabled more people to age with a wide range of chronic conditions and survive conditions that may have been fatal to previous generations. They are better informed than previous generations, which influences their desire to be actively engaged in their health care. An understanding of the general realities of the older population can assist nurses in preparing for some of the challenges of gerontological nursing.

Objectives

In this chapter you will learn to:

1. Describe characteristics of today's older population in regard to:
   - Life expectancy
   - Marital status
   - Health status
   - Income and employment
   - Education
   - Diversity

LIFE EXPECTANCY

The average number of years that an individual can anticipate to live is referred to as *life expectancy*. Less than a century ago, the life expectancy in the United States was 54.1 years; today it is 77.9 years (Table 1.1). The rising life expectancy has resulted in an increase in the number of persons age 65 years and older, who now represent 12% of the total population. The aging of the Baby Boomers (people born between 1946 and 1964) will substantially increase the older population between now and 2030, causing them to represent 20% of the total population.

FAST FACTS in a NUTSHELL

There are differences in life expectancy based on gender and race. Women live longer than men and White people live longer than Black individuals. In fact, life expectancy among the Black population has declined due to an increase in deaths from homicide and AIDS.

In addition to more people reaching old age, they are living longer when they do. Approximately 40% of the older population is over age 85 and the number of centenarians is increasing.

Living longer means little if those extra years are riddled with disease and disability. A reasonable goal for this population is to reduce the years in which health and function are impaired. The delaying or compressing of the years in which the older adult experiences illness and decline is referred to as *compression of morbidity*.

TABLE 1.1 Life Expectancy in the United States

Year	Total U.S. Population	White Population			Black Population		
		Total	Men	Women	Total	Men	Women
2007	77.0	78.4	79.5	80.8	75.6	70.0	76.8
2010 (projected)	78.5	79.0	76.1	81.8	74.5	70.9	77.8

From Centers for Disease Control and Prevention, National Center for Health Statistics (2011). Health, United States, 2010: With Special Feature on Death and Dying. Table 22, Life expectancy at birth by race and sex. Hyattsville, MD.

MARITAL STATUS

Due to their longer life expectancy and tendency to marry men older than themselves, most older women are widowed, while most older men have living spouses. Older women are more likely to live alone.

================= *FAST FACTS in a NUTSHELL*

Because most older women have outlived their spouses, they are less likely to have an available caregiver to assist them in their homes. Additionally, as they have a longer life expectancy, they are also more likely to reach the years in which they will need assistance to manage their daily care. It is important to ask specific questions during the assessment to uncover the need for assistance, particularly as these women, who may have long put the needs of their families and households ahead of their own, may not share their personal care needs.

HEALTH STATUS

Chronic conditions are a major health challenge for older individuals (Table 1.2). Most older adults have at least one chronic condition; having multiple chronic conditions is not uncommon. The effects of these conditions (e.g., pain, reduced mobility, impaired communication) can significantly affect quality of life for older adults.

Acute conditions are of lower incidence among the older population; however, they often result in more complications, longer periods of recovery, and higher rates of mortality in this population.

Heart disease is the leading cause of death among persons age 65 and older. Other leading causes, in order of incidence, are: cancer; chronic lower respiratory disease; cerebrovascular disease; Alzheimer's disease; diabetes mellitus; influenza and pneumonia; nephritis, nephrotic syndrome and nephrosis; accidents; and septicemia.

Less than 5% of older adults are in a nursing home or assisted living community at any given time, although approximately one fourth of this population will spend some time in these facilities during their lifetimes.

TABLE 1.2 Leading Chronic Conditions Affecting Population Age 65 and Older
1. Arthritis
2. High blood pressure
3. Hearing impairments
4. Heart conditions
5. Visual impairments (including cataracts)
6. Deformities or orthopedic impairments
7. Diabetes mellitus
8. Chronic sinusitis
9. Hay fever, allergic rhinitis (without asthma)
10. Varicose veins

From Centers for Disease Control and Prevention, Chronic Disease Prevention and Health Promotion, www.cdc.gov/chronicdisease/index.htm, accessed 11/14/12.

INCOME

Although the poverty rate has been declining for older adults, they are hardly without financial challenges. A majority of older adults depend on Social Security for more than half of their income. They have a higher median net worth than other age groups, but this is because of the equity in their homes. Unless older adults sell their homes or obtain a reverse mortgage, they may be asset rich but cash poor.

Rising cost of living is causing more Baby Boomers to re-enter or remain in the labor force than in the past. Their continued employment is also influenced by their desire and ability to stay engaged in work longer than previous generations.

EDUCATION

The educational level of each generation of older adults has increased. Growing numbers of this population hold college degrees. Nurses can expect older persons to be better informed and engaged health care consumers.

DIVERSITY

It is estimated that between 2000 and 2050, the non-Hispanic White older population will decrease from 84% to 64%. By 2020, one in four older adults will belong to a minority racial or ethnic group (Administration on Aging, 2012; U.S. Census Bureau, 2012). During this time the Hispanic elderly, the fastest growing segment of the U.S. population, are projected to significantly increase, to constitute 20% of the total older population. The lower life expectancy of the Black population accounts for a smaller percentage of Blacks represented among the elderly; however, the older Black population will grow from 8% to 11% between now and 2050. Interestingly, once a Black individual reaches the seventh decade of life, life expectancy begins to be similar to older White persons. The Asian population, representing individuals from countries such as China, Japan, the Philippines, Korea, Vietnam, and Cambodia, represents approximately 4% of the older adult population. Only 8% of the Native American population is older than 65 years of age, representing less than 1% of all older adults; however, they are one of the fastest growing minorities of the older population.

FAST FACTS in a NUTSHELL

Considerable diversity can exist among people of the same faith, ethnicity, race, or sexual orientation. Learning about the individual is essential.

In addition to racial and ethnic diversity, consideration must be given to the sexual diversity among older adults. As much as 10% of the population identifies itself as lesbian, gay, bisexual, or transgender (LGBT), and this population is projected to double by 2030. The awareness and needs of the older LGBT population has been given so little consideration that it is referred to as a largely invisible population (Fredriksen-Goldsen et al., 2011). Sensitivity to this group has been growing. AARP has created an online LGBT community, the American Society on Aging has an LGBT Aging Issues Network, and The Joint Commission has added respect for sexual orientation to the rights of residents of assisted living communities and skilled nursing homes. In addition, Services and Advocacy for Gay, Lesbian, Bisexual, & Transgender Elders (SAGE) and the Movement Advancement Project (MAP) have been aggressively addressing policy and regulatory changes that are needed to address the needs of this population.

Just as we wouldn't assume all 25 year olds or all 40 year olds to be similar in terms of profile, health status, and nursing needs, we cannot make generalizations about the older population. Greater numbers of people representing minorities comprise the older population. Medical advancements have allowed more people to survive to late life with complex health conditions and growing numbers stay active, healthy, and functional in advanced years. Easy access to information has equipped aging individuals to be more informed consumers than previous generations and to challenge their health care providers. In addition, older adults may demand health services that enable them to look and feel young well into their senior years. Nurses will be challenged to provide state-of-the-art evidence-based care, tailored to meet the needs of a highly diverse population and to employ strategies to empower them to be active participants in their care.

2

The Nursing Process in Geriatric Care

Nurses have a unique role in geriatric care in that they are involved in patients' total needs: physical, mental, emotional, social, and spiritual. By using a systematic approach called the nursing process, nurses assess patients' status, identify needs, plan care, coordinate care activities with other disciplines, implement activities to promote wellness and manage health conditions, and evaluate the effectiveness of plans and activities. Nurses' competencies in performing these activities and their presence in virtually every care setting enable them to demonstrate significant leadership in geriatric care.

Objectives

In this chapter you will learn to:

1. Identify sources of data that contribute to the assessment process
2. Describe factors that can interfere with the assessment process
3. Describe three general assessment techniques
4. Outline a method for organizing assessment data
5. Identify tools that are available for various components of the assessment
6. Describe factors that affect patients' self-care capacity
7. List characteristics of effective care plans
8. Describe methods for engaging patients in assessment, care planning, and care activities

PREPARING FOR THE ASSESSMENT

Assessment is the process of collecting and analyzing data. During the process of assessing older adults, a variety of subjective and objective data is collected and interpreted. Data can be obtained from:

- Medical records and other documents
- The patient
- The patient's family, friends
- Caregivers (formal and informal)
- Other disciplines

A comprehensive assessment is often done when the patient is admitted to the caregiving service and at specific time intervals thereafter. As a significant amount of information is collected and examination and testing procedures performed, the assessment experience can be tiring for the older patient; therefore, the assessment may need to be completed during several sessions so as not to tire the patient. In addition, many of today's older adults have had limited experience being interviewed and sharing information about bodily functions, feelings, family relationships, and other issues, so an explanation of the reason this information is being requested, how it benefits care, and that it will be held in confidence will prove helpful. The patient should be advised that he or she can ask questions or seek clarification for terms or questions that are not understood.

FAST FACTS in a NUTSHELL

Slower responses, poorer memory, and a longer life history can cause assessments to require more time to complete for older adults than younger ones. Adequate time should be planned, and, if necessary, the assessment should be broken into several shorter sessions rather than completed during one lengthy one.

Memory may be poor in older persons, and special hints to trigger recall may be needed. For example, instead of asking patients if they have any allergies, asking if any drugs, lotions, materials, or food have ever caused them to become sick or develop a rash could yield better information.

It is useful to determine if hearing deficits are present. Ignored questions or inappropriate responses could be associated with impaired hearing.

Environmental factors can facilitate or impair the assessment, such as:

- *Room temperature.* Older adults' increased sensitivity to lower environmental temperatures could reduce their comfort and attentiveness if the room used for the assessment is too cool. Rooms that are too cool are not only a concern in winter months, but in the summer, as well, when air conditioners are set on low temperatures. A room temperature of 75°F (24°C) is usually adequate for most older adults; however, as individuals vary, it is useful to ask about the appropriateness of the room temperature.
- *Glare.* Cataracts are problems affecting most older adults and result in glare being more bothersome. Adjusting window coverings and patient seating to prevent direct sunlight from shining on the patient's face and using lighting sources that are indirect and soft (e.g., not fluorescent lighting) facilitate patient comfort.
- *Distractions.* Noise and heavy traffic can prevent patients from hearing and focusing during the assessment. A quiet area separated from other activity will reduce distractions and promote a sense of privacy. If the assessment must be conducted in a semi-private room, pull the curtain and position yourself on the side of the bed farthest away from the roommate's bed so that the patient is less aware of the presence of the roommate.
- *Access to bathrooms.* Older adults need to void more frequently than younger adults, so conducting the assessment in an area in which a bathroom is easily accessible, and offering the patient the opportunity to use the bathroom before beginning the assessment, are helpful measures.

METHODS OF ASSESSING

To plan comprehensive care, it is essential to have insight into the physical, emotional, and mental function and socioeconomic status of the patient. The complexity and wealth of information that each older adult possesses demands that multiple techniques be used in the assessment process. Most assessment techniques involve the skills of *observation, interview,* and *examination.*

========================= *FAST FACTS in a NUTSHELL*

The patient's general appearance can reveal much about self-concept, self-care capacity, mental status, and cultural practices.

Observation

Observation refers to the deliberate use of all the senses to gather information. Every nurse-patient contact can afford the opportunity to observe for general status and changes. As some patients, such as those with dementias, may not accurately report problems and symptoms, keen observation assists in identifying problems in an early stage. Observe:

- General appearance
- Areas of discoloration, cuts, bruises, or sores
- Posture and body movement
- Eye contact and body language
- Quality, appropriateness, and loudness of speech
- Unusual sounds, such as wheezes, intestinal gurgling, or loose-fitting dentures
- Reaction to touch
- Grip of handshake
- Odors

========================= *FAST FACTS in a NUTSHELL*

Noting odors can be beneficial in identifying other problems and risks. The excessive use of cologne or strong body odors could indicate the patient's poor sense of smell, which may trigger safety concerns as the patient may not detect smoke or gas leaks in the home. Breath odor could be related to poor oral hygiene, lung abscesses, alcohol consumption, and infections of the oral cavity. A sweet, fruity breath odor usually is associated with increased acetone levels from diabetic acidosis. Uremic acidosis gives the breath an odor of stale urine.

Interview

The validity and depth of information the patient is willing to provide is strongly influenced by the degree of trust in the nurse conducting the interview, so the establishment of rapport is crucial. Some measures that will facilitate the interview process are to:

- Ensure the patient is comfortable
- Provide a distance of approximately 4 feet between the patient and you
- Advise the patient of the purpose of the interview and examination, and how long it is expected to last
- Use language appropriate to the patient; avoid medical jargon
- Plan questions in terms of content and style
- Listen
- Pay attention to the content of what is being said, as well as the tone and body language that accompanies it
- Summarize and validate information obtained

FAST FACTS in a NUTSHELL

Different styles of questions are effective for eliciting different types of information. Closed-ended questions that are direct and elicit short answers are useful when concise, nonexplanatory information is sought (e.g., Did you refill your prescription? How long have you been using a hearing aid?). Open-ended questions encourage discussion and often yield information and insight into the patient's thinking and behavior that otherwise may have been missed. Examples of open-ended questions include: How would you describe your pain? What are your most important concerns?

Examination

Assessment of mood and cognition begins upon first observation of the patient and continues through the interview by noting poor grooming and inappropriate responses, affect, body language, and general behavior. Several mental status examination tools are available to guide a standardized assessment of mood and cognition (see Box 1). The specific steps to assessing mental status are discussed in Chapter 11.

Physical examination consists of collecting data through the use of:

- *Inspection:* visualizing the body for normality of structure and function
- *Auscultation:* using a stethoscope to hear sounds within the body
- *Percussion:* Determining the intensity, pitch, quality, and duration of sounds created by tapping the body surface
- *Palpation:* Touching and manipulating body parts for their size, temperature, texture, and mobility

Other chapters in this text will offer instructions pertaining to the assessment of specific systems.

There are many evidence-based assessment tools available that can be used in assessing older adults. Some are general and others targeted at a specific issue, such as incontinence, pressure ulcers, or oral health. The Hartford Institute for Geriatric Nursing website includes many of the popular tools used in assessing older adults and is a useful resource to explore (see Box 1).

Box 2.1   Assessment Tools Available Through the Hartford Institute for Geriatric Nursing *Try This* Series
www.hartfordign.org/practice/try_this/

SPICES: An Overall Assessment Tool of Older Adults
Katz Index of Independence in Activities of Daily Living (ADL)
Mental Status Assessment of Older Adults: The Mini-Co
The Geriatric Depression Scale (GDS)
Predicting Pressure Ulcer Risk
The Pittsburgh Sleep Quality Index (PSQI)

(continued)

ORGANIZING DATA COLLECTION

During a comprehensive assessment of an older adult a considerable amount of information can be obtained, which could prove overwhelming and difficult to use. Organizing data will facilitate its use in care planning and delivery. Box 2.2 outlines useful data to obtain through the assessment and a framework for organizing it.

Box 2.2   Assessment Components and Framework

Name _____

Sex _____ Race/Ethnicity _____

Date of birth: After asking date of birth, follow with a question such as, *"That makes you how old?"* not only to validate data, but to also gain insight into long- and short-term memory.

Languages spoken: This may be useful in identifying the need for an interpreter if the patient is not fluent in the English language. Also, under stressful conditions, a bilingual patient may resort to his or her native tongue, so it is useful to be aware of the language that could be used.

Religion: Not only the type of religion, but specific name of the church, temple, or synagogue, and the patient's relationship to it are useful. Often, religious organizations provide assistance and visitation to older adults. In addition, special diets and practices consistent with religious and cultural beliefs should be explored.

Education: As important as the patient's formal education is functional ability. Asking questions such as, *"Do you read the daily papers?"* and,*"Was the insurance form difficult to complete?"* can offer insights.

Contact person: This is not always the next of kin, but any significant person in the elder's life.

Employment status: As increasing numbers of older adults are remaining and returning to the workforce, it is useful to learn if the patient is employed and if it is by choice or necessity. The type of occupation can offer clues into possible occupation-related diseases.

(continued)

Finances: Review income and expenses (unless done by the social worker).

Health insurance: Knowing the type of insurance can help in understanding the services that may and may not be reimbursed.

Marital status: Ask the spouse's or partner's age, health, and occupation. If widowed, ask when the death occurred, resulting lifestyle adjustments, and current feelings about death.

Children: Obtain the children's names, locations, and ages. Discussions of relationships with children can help determine the extent to which they may be a source of support or distress to the patient.

Support systems: Ask about relatives, friends, neighbors, or professionals who play a significant role in the patient's life.

Housing: Ask about the type of housing, number of levels and stairs, presence of kitchen facilities, location of bathroom, source of heat, general condition, nearest neighbor, and ability to maintain and afford.

Living arrangements: Review the members of the household. Some older adults have grandchildren living with them, for whom they provide care and support.

Household responsibilities: Review the type of tasks for which the patient is responsible.

Pets: Determine types of animals with which the patient has contact, ability to care for a pet (physically and economically), and the role of the pet in the elder's life.

Social/leisure activities: Review the types of activities in which the patient engages and enjoys.

Functional ability: Determine the patient's ability to fulfill activities of daily living (eating, dressing, bathing, grooming, walking, transferring, climbing stairs, communicating, and toileting) and instrumental activities of daily living (using the phone, taking medications, handling finances, preparing meals, doing laundry, housekeeping, home maintenance, using transportation, leisure activities). Explore how deficits are managed.

Ethnic/religious practices: Review practices that can affect activities, dress code, diet, relationships, and health care beliefs.

Self-appraisal of health: Ask the patient to describe how he or she is feeling or evaluate his or her health.

(continued)

Box 2.2 Assessment Components and Framework (*continued*)

Health practices: Ask the patient to describe practices to stay healthy, such as taking supplements, exercising, and getting regular check-ups.

Allergies: Give the patient specific clues to trigger memory of allergies, such as skin rashes, hives, nausea, fainting, or headaches associated with specific foods, drugs, animals, or chemicals.

Known diseases: Ask the patient to describe health conditions, how and when they were diagnosed, and how they are managed.

Resources used: List all health and social resources used, including nature and frequency of contact.

Medications: List the names of all prescription and over-the-counter drugs used. (Ideally, the patient should be encouraged to bring all medications used to the examination.)

Diet: List how, when, and what the patient eats. Explore food preferences and restrictions.

Voiding pattern: Ask the patient to describe frequency, amount, continence, and any problem associated with urination.

Bowel elimination: Ask the patient to describe the frequency, pattern, continence, and characteristics of bowel movements.

Sleep and rest pattern: Determine the patient's usual bedtime and rising time. Explore interruptions to sleep. Describe the number, length, and pattern of naps.

Sexual history: Inquire about sexual interest, function, and problems.

Complaints: Ask about symptoms and concerns.

Goals: Ask the patient what he or she hopes to achieve or his or her desires.

Mental status: Describe level of consciousness, cognition, memory, and judgment. Ask about changes in mental function that have been noted. Include results of mental status tests.

Mood: Note evidence of depression, anxiety, paranoia, and other emotional symptoms. Ask about thoughts of suicide, satisfaction with life, views of self, and any concerns.

Systems review: Document findings identified during the assessment of each system.

Other: Describe any other significant findings.

Health care organizations often develop and/or utilize assessment tools that address their specific care focus. The *minimum data set* (MDS) used in nursing homes is an example of a tool specific to that setting. The MDS is a federally mandated assessment process for residents in Medicaid- and Medicare-certified nursing homes. (The full tool can be reviewed at the Centers for Medicare and Medicaid website.)

FACTORS AFFECTING SELF-CARE CAPACITY

During the assessment, health conditions and care needs may be identified. These problems and needs will help to guide the care plan components and priorities. However, in addition to identifying the problem or need, it is important to determine the patient's capacity for self-care so that specific actions can be planned. Factors that affect self-care capacity that are useful to assess include:

- *Functional ability:* Impairments in the ability to process information and not knowing how to appropriately respond, move the body, and have the body function in a normal manner can impair the ability to engage in self-care. In addition to physical and mental abilities, socioeconomic abilities can influence self-care, as can occur when a person cannot afford a healthy diet or prescribed medications.

FAST FACTS in a NUTSHELL

As plans and actions differ depending on the cause of the self-care deficit, identifying the factors responsible is an important part of the assessment.

- *Competencies:* Knowledge, skills, and experience contribute to satisfactorily fulfilling self-care demands. For example, a person's lack of understanding as to what constitutes a healthy diet and competency in preparing meals can result in consumption of an unhealthy diet from the local fast-food restaurant.

- *Motivation:* An individual may have no physical, mental, competency, or financial limitations that prevent engagement in self-care, but may lack the motivation to perform these activities. For example, a woman may see no need to bathe and get out of her bathrobe for days if she has no social activity outside the home. Or, an older man may feel that the stress and effort of exercising isn't worth the ability to remain ambulatory and choose to use a wheelchair instead.

TEAM INVOLVEMENT

To understand the complete profile of patients it is useful to have the input of various disciplines that may be involved with the patients. The assessments of various physicians, therapists, and pharmacists, along with the insights of nursing assistants and other team members, contribute to the understanding of all aspects of patients. In addition, team collaboration aids in directing care planning by ensuring all needs have been identified and appropriate actions planned.

CARE PLANNING

Due to the extensive life histories and prevalence of health conditions in older adults, a considerable amount of information is often collected during the assessment. Careful review of the information is crucial to identifying the most significant and urgent issues that need to be addressed. The identified problems and needs are prioritized and used to develop goals. Some characteristics of well-developed goals are that they are:

- *Statements of what the patient will achieve.* Goals state the desired outcomes for the patient, not what the staff will do. A goal that states "Patient will ambulate at least 50 feet BID" reflects the goal for the patient more than a goal stating "Staff will ambulate patient daily."
- *Measurable.* The goals must be objective and specific enough to enable different people to achieve similar conclusions when evaluating if the goal was met. For example, a goal that states the patient will "lose weight" can create difficulty in

evaluation, as one nurse can think the goal is achieved if the resident loses 2 pounds per month while another may feel a weight loss of 10 pounds per month is insufficient. A goal that the patient will "lose 10 pounds per month for the next 3 months" offers specific outcomes that can be evaluated.

Interventions are then developed for each goal. These must reflect actions that can be realistically performed. For example, stating that a patient will be checked every 15 minutes may seem impressive, but if the reality is that patients cannot be monitored that frequently in the given setting, that action is not achievable and offers little useful direction to staff. Further, should a fall or complication occur when this action was on the care plan and the staff was not checking on the patient every 15 minutes, the charge could be made that the staff was negligent because they failed to provide an action that they recognized as necessary.

FAST FACTS in a NUTSHELL

Nurses utilize a variety of approaches to assist patients in achieving goals, which can include teaching, coaching, counseling, monitoring, coordinating services, partially assisting, or completely doing a task for the patient. It is important that the approach planned be stated as specifically as possible to guide the staff.

Although the nurse guides and coordinates care planning activities, ideally every discipline involved with the patient's care participates in the development of the care plan. To the degree possible, patients and, upon their consent, significant others should actively participate in the care plan. The goals and planned actions should be reviewed with the patient, not only to advise the patient of the plan, but also to offer the patient an opportunity to describe agreement or the lack thereof.

The time frame for completing the care plan varies depending on the site. In a nursing home, a care plan is usually required to be developed within 1 week after the completion of the assessment and revised whenever there is a change in status. In acute care settings, a care plan may be developed within the first several hours to guide care of an unstable or critically ill patient.

The care plan needs to be revised when there is a change in status. When changes are made to the care plan, the original statements on the plan should not be erased or obliterated, as they may need to be reviewed at a later time. The change should be highlighted or have a line drawn through and the new information added. All revisions to the care plan need to be communicated to all caregivers.

ENGAGING THE PATIENT

To the maximum degree possible, patients need to be active participants in all aspects of their care. Encouraging them to express concerns, demonstrating patience, and listening to what is communicated assists in obtaining realistic, thorough insights into patients' status and function that can promote accurate, comprehensive assessments. Reviewing with patients the problems and needs that have been identified and potential interventions to assist with them ensures that plans address the issues of concern to patients and equips them with an understanding of expected care activities. Ensuring that patients participate in care activities to the fullest extent of their abilities and offering them maximum choices in the manner in which these activities are conducted promote their independence and compliance, as well as demonstrate respect for their right to determine their life and care actions.

FAST FACTS in a NUTSHELL

Care not only needs to be patient-centered, but also, to the maximum extent possible, patient-directed. This may result in dietary, activity, schedule, treatment, and other choices being less than textbook perfect; however, it honors the right of competent older adults to control their lives.

Normalcy and Disease
in Late Life

3

Cardiovascular System

The cardiovascular system's role in delivering oxygen and nutrients to all body organs, and transporting carbon dioxide and other wastes away from them, causes the cardiovascular system to have a profound role in ensuring the body's homeostasis. The status of this system, therefore, significantly affects health and functional capacity. A variety of cardiovascular changes do occur with age, which results from both normal aging and other factors. As the prevalence of cardiovascular conditions increases with age and can present atypically, careful assessment is crucial to ensure timely identification and treatment. In addition, education related to lifestyle practices that contribute to cardiovascular health is important to assisting aging individuals in reducing risks.

Objectives

In this chapter you will learn to:

1. Identify common age-related changes to the cardiovascular system
2. Outline the components of a cardiovascular system nursing assessment

3. Identify symptoms associated with the following cardiovascular conditions:
   - Heart failure
   - Hypertension
   - Angina
   - Myocardial infarction
   - Hyperlipidemia
   - Varicose veins
4. Describe nursing actions to support the treatment of the following cardiovascular conditions:
   - Heart failure
   - Hypertension
   - Angina
   - Myocardial infarction
   - Hyperlipidemia
   - Varicose veins
5. Describe general measures to promote cardiovascular health in older adults

AGE-RELATED CHANGES

Some of the cardiovascular changes experienced by older adults that were once considered normal outcomes of aging have been found to be the result of pathological conditions. For example, there once was the belief that heart size changed with age; this was later found to be associated with cardiac disease or atrophy from insufficient activity levels. Among the cardiovascular changes that are attributed to aging are:

- Slight left ventricular hypertrophy
- Enlargement of the left atrium
- Dilation and elongation of the aorta
- Thickening and rigidity of the atrioventricular valves, interfering with contraction of the heart
- Systolic and diastolic murmurs associated with incomplete valve closure
- Irritability of the myocardium, leading to sinus arrhythmia and extra systolic sinus bradycardia
- Changes in resting electrocardiogram due to reduction in pacemaker and conduction cells

- High prevalence of extra heart sound due to atrial contractions in diastole, S4
- Prolonged isometric contraction phase and relaxation time of left ventricle
- More time needed for completion of diastolic filling and systolic emptying cycle
- Increased systolic blood pressure due to impaired baroreceptor function and increased peripheral resistance
- Impaired regulation of blood pressure due to impaired baroreceptor function, leading to postural hypotension

Most older adults adapt to these changes by adjusting activities (e.g., taking an elevator instead of stairs and pacing activities); therefore, daily activities typically are not significantly affected. The changes are most noted when an unusual demand is placed on the heart, such as engaging in exercise or experiencing emotional stress. Tachycardia may be experienced for a longer period of time than would occur in a younger adult.

ASSESSMENT CONSIDERATIONS

Assessment of the cardiovascular system begins with observation of:

- *General coloring:* Note pallor
- *Energy level:* Note posture, speed of responses, activity level, evidence of fatigue
- *Respirations:* Observe expansion of lungs during inspiration, bilateral symmetry of lung movement, dyspnea, rate and regularity of respirations
- *Nail condition:* Inspect for clubbing (associated with advanced cardiac disease), thickness, dryness, response to blanching (circulatory insufficiency can delay return of pink color to nails after blanching)
- *Extremities:* Note varicosities, discoloration, edema, hair loss (which can indicate poor circulation)
- *Mental status:* Altered cognition and level of consciousness can occur with insufficient cerebral circulation

The interview uses structured questions to identify lifestyle practices, symptoms, and risks that influence cardiovascular health. Specific questions could include:

- How often do you exercise and what type of exercises do you do?
- What vitamin and herbal supplements do you take?
- Could you give me an example of your typical daily diet?
- Do you drink alcoholic beverages? If so, how much and how often?
- What type of things do you do to promote health?
- What medications, prescribed and over-the-counter, are you taking?
- Do you have any difficulty or have you had any changes in your ability to walk or stand?
- Are you able to bathe and dress yourself?
- Are you able to get out and shop, attend church/temple, and engage in social activities?
- Do you ever feel dizzy or lightheaded?*
- Do you ever have pain or strange feelings in your chest, shoulder, or arms?*
- Do you have dull headaches or nosebleeds (these may be indicative of hypertension)?*
- Have you noticed any changes in your thinking, memory, or mental clearness?*
- Does exercise or activity cause you to get extremely tired, short of breath, or have palpitations?*
- Do your feet and ankles swell as the day goes on? Do you find that your fingers swell as the day goes on?*
- Do you bruise easily?*

Strive to put the patient at ease during the interview and address any questions or concerns that may be expressed. Then, prepare the patient for the physical examination. Conduct the examination as follows:

- Starting at the head, inspect the body. Note distended vessels, varicosities, areas of redness, pallor, cyanosis, lesions, edema, and bruises.

If positive response is given, ask about onset, frequency, duration, management, and characteristics of symptoms.

- Assess apical and radial pulse. The normal rate should range between 60 and 100 beats per minute. Keep in mind that some tachycardia can be present due to the activity that the patient engaged in hours before the examination and the stress of the examination. If tachycardia is detected, reassess at a later time.
- Measure blood pressure with the patient seated comfortably with both feet on the floor. It should be measured at least twice with a 5-minutes rest period between each measurement. Obtaining blood pressure in a lying, sitting, and standing position is useful to detect postural hypotension. Postural drops greater than 20 mmHg are significant.
- Auscultate the heart. Note thrills and bruits.
- Assess pulse bilaterally at these sites:
  - *Temporal pulse*—the only palpable artery of the head, located anterior to the ear, overlying the temporal bone; normally appears tortuous
  - *Brachial pulse*—located in the groove between the biceps and triceps; usually palpated if arterial insufficiency is suspected
  - *Radial pulse*—branching from the brachial artery, the radial artery extends from the forearm to the wrist on the radial side and is palpated on the flexor surface of the wrist laterally
  - *Ulnar pulse*—also branching from the brachial artery, the ulnar artery extends from the forearm to the wrist on the ulnar side and is palpated on the flexor surface of the wrist medially; usually palpated if arterial insufficiency is suspected
  - *Femoral pulse*—the femoral artery is palpated at the inguinal ligament midway between the anterosuperior iliac spine and the pubic tubercle
  - *Popliteal pulse*—located behind the knee; the popliteal artery is the continuation of the femoral artery. Having the patient flex the knee during palpitation can aid in locating this pulse
  - *Posterior tibial pulse*—palpable behind and below the medial malleolus
  - *Dorsalis pedis pulse*—palpated at the groove between the first two tendons on the medial side of the dorsum of the foot; this and the posterior tibial pulse can be congenitally absent

- Rate pulses on a scale from 0 to 4 (often, a stick figure is used to document the quality of pulses at different locations):
    - 0 = no pulse
    - 1 = thready, easily obliterated pulse
    - 2 = pulse difficult to palpate and easily obliterated
    - 3 = normal pulse
    - 4 = strong, bounding pulse, not obliterated with pressure
- Determine if the patient has had a recent electrocardiogram and blood work, including C-reactive protein (CRP) screening (CRP is a marker of inflammation that is a stronger predictor of cardiovascular events than low-density lipoprotein [LDL] cholesterol). The American Heart Association and the Centers for Disease Control and Prevention have recommended CRP screening for persons at moderate risk of heart disease (Ridker, 2003).

Any unusual findings should be explored and described fully in the documentation.

CONDITIONS

Improvements in preventive measures, diagnostic testing, and treatment have resulted in lower death rates from cardiovascular conditions. Despite these advancements, cardiovascular disease is a significant health problem and remains the leading cause of death for the population age 65 years and older. Effective nursing interventions make a significant contribution to helping older adults avoid complications and live a high-quality life with cardiovascular conditions.

FAST FACTS in a NUTSHELL

Cardiovascular disease affects and kills significantly more women than breast cancer, yet women often are unaware of symptoms of cardiovascular conditions or delay seeking attention when symptoms do appear. Nurses need to educate aging women about their risk for cardiovascular disease and symptoms warranting attention, and ask about symptoms during every assessment.

Heart Failure

Heart failure (HF) not only significantly increases with age, with most of the people affected being over age 65 years, but is also the most common cause of hospitalizations for the older population. As it has been found that about half of these admissions could have been prevented (Jurgens, Hoke, Byrnes, & Riegel, 2009), nursing actions to teach patients preventive measures, monitoring of medication compliance, and early detection of symptoms can reduce the risk of hospitalizations and complications.

Persons at highest risk for developing HF include obese individuals and those with hypertension, coronary artery disease, myocardial infarction, diabetes mellitus, and valvular heart disease. It is more common for men to develop HF than women, although women with diabetes mellitus are at high risk. Related risk factors that can contribute to this problem include cigarette smoking, sedentary lifestyle, dyslipidemia, sleep-disordered breathing, chronic renal disease, stress, amphetamine and cocaine use, alcohol abuse, and chronic use of nonsteroidal anti-inflammatory drugs and thiazolidinediones. These risk factors, along with nonadherence to the treatment plan and acute infection, also can contribute to readmission for HF after the initial hospitalization.

Symptoms of HF are consistent with the presence of pulmonary congestion and reduced cardiac output, and include:

- Dyspnea on exertion (the most common finding)
- Confusion or worsening of dementia-related confusion, agitation
- Tachycardia
- Weight gain
- Bilateral ankle edema
- Insomnia, nighttime wandering
- Depression
- Anorexia, nausea
- Weakness
- Shortness of breath, orthopnea
- Wheezing
- Moist crackles heard on auscultation

Specific questions about dietary intake should be asked, as high sodium intake could contribute to fluid overload. In addition to asking about the addition of salt to food, it is useful to ask about specific high-sodium foods that may be consumed, such as lunch meats, canned foods, snack foods, and fast foods.

A review of prescription and over-the-counter medications is included in the assessment. Patients may have been prescribed diuretics that they are not taking, which contributed to their HF. The reasons for not taking diuretics as prescribed needs to be explored, as different causes (e.g., confusion as to how to take the drug, inability to afford the prescription, desire to avoid frequent trips to the bathroom) warrant different nursing interventions.

FAST FACTS in a NUTSHELL

Although similar assessment methods are used for assessing for HF in older adults as would be used for adults of other ages, consideration should be given to the possibility that other conditions could cause similar symptoms—dyspnea may not be evident due to reduced activity levels, and older adults may not report symptoms, erroneously believing such symptoms are normal at their age. This challenges nurses to ask about specific symptoms and to review the patient's health history carefully.

The presence of symptoms consistent with HF needs to be reported to the physician promptly. The history and physical examination confirm the diagnosis. A 12-lead electrocardiogram (ECG) and chest x-ray are part of the examination. Laboratory tests typically include complete blood count, serum electrolytes, lipid profile, blood urea nitrogen, serum creatinine, fasting blood glucose, glycosylated hemoglobin A1c (HbA1c), liver function tests, thyroid stimulating hormone, and urinalysis. Renal function is an important consideration in the assessment because altered renal function in older adults with HF can cause life-threatening hyperkalemia when these individuals are given certain cardiovascular drugs, such as angiotensin-converting enzyme (ACE) inhibitors, angiotensin II receptor blockers, and aldosterone antagonists (Poggio, Grancelli, & Miruka, 2010).

The initial treatment goals for the patient with HF are to identify and correct the underlying cause, alleviate symptoms, and improve circulation. ACE inhibitors, beta blockers, digitalis, diuretics, and a reduction in sodium intake typically are prescribed. Initially, bed rest may be recommended, with the patient being allowed to sit in a chair next to the bed. Complete bedrest is not recommended due to the risk for thrombosis and pulmonary congestion. The patient's response to activity should be noted, with particular attention to fatigue, dyspnea, pallor, and changes in vital signs.

FAST FACTS in a NUTSHELL

It is important to assess vital signs during various levels of activity in the patient with HF. A decrease in blood pressure and increase in pulse are signs of reduced cardiac output.

Nursing actions for the patient with HF will include:

- Administering medications as prescribed; instructing the patient about medications that will be used for ongoing management of the condition.
- Administering oxygen as ordered (oxygen may be contraindicated or prescribed at lower levels for the patient with chronic hypoxia).
- Instructing the patient on fluid and sodium restrictions that are ordered.
- Observing changes in vital signs, weight, and mental status. (Confusion, agitation, restlessness, and altered levels of consciousness could indicate reduced cerebral circulation.) Note edema, dyspnea, loss of appetite, and other symptoms.
- Protecting skin from pressure ulcers.
- Elevating and supporting extremities while the patient is sitting in a chair.
- Scheduling activities to allow rest periods between activities.
- Applying antiembolism stockings as ordered.
- Assessing the patient's learning needs and teaching measures for management of the condition accordingly. Advise the patient and/or caregiver to note and report symptoms such as edema, dizziness, weight gain of 3 pounds or more, increased fatigue, chest or abdominal pain, bleeding, bruising, or shortness of breath with activities that were previously tolerated.

Hypertension

Hypertension refers to a systolic blood pressure ≥140 mmHg and a diastolic blood pressure ≥90 mmHg. More than half of all older adults have hypertension, with women having a higher prevalence than men.

The increased incidence of hypertension with age causes this to be the most prevalent cardiovascular disease of older adults.

═══════════════════════════ *FAST FACTS in a NUTSHELL*

Systolic blood pressure continues to rise throughout life, unlike diastolic blood pressure, which rises until age 50 and then stays the same or slightly falls. Despite a normal diastolic blood pressure, treatment may be needed if systolic blood pressure is elevated (National Institutes of Health, 2004).

The initial blood pressure reading should be obtained in both arms with a properly sized cuff. To use the auscultatory method for blood pressure measurement, place the cuff on the arm, palpate the radial pulse, inflate the cuff, and identify the point at which the pulse disappears. Future blood pressure measurements should be done by inflating to at least 30 mmHg above that point. When assessing blood pressure, consider the activities that preceded the assessment if the blood pressure is found to be high. Unusual activity or the stress involved in preparing for a visit to the health care provider can cause a rise in blood pressure. If an elevated blood pressure is found, allow the patient to rest for 10 minutes and retake the blood pressure. Obtain the blood pressure in lying, sitting, and standing positions. Postural drops greater than 20 mmHg are significant.

Ask about symptoms of hypertension, which can include confusion, epistaxis, dull headache, impaired memory, and a slow tremor.

═══════════════════════════ *FAST FACTS in a NUTSHELL*

Nurses should teach, assist, and coach patients with learning yoga, biofeedback, meditation, and relaxation exercises as measures to manage mild hypertension.

A variety of treatment options can be employed for the treatment of hypertension. As antihypertensive medications can have many unintended effects (e.g., orthostatic hypotension, sedation, depression, delirium, constipation, erectile dysfunction), these drugs should be used only when absolutely necessary and when nonpharmacological methods have proven ineffective.

A diet low in sodium and rich in whole-grain foods is useful in preventing and managing hypertension. Instruct the patient in dietary practices or refer to a dietician.

Box 3.1 describes some of the antihypertensive medications that could be prescribed, as well as the related nursing interventions.

Box 3. I Safe Use of Antihypertensive Medications

ACE inhibitors
(Include benazepril, captopril, enalapril, fosinopril, lisinopril, moexipril, perindopril, quinapril, ramipril, and trandolapril)

These drugs are popular initial agents in the treatment of hypertension and tend to be well-tolerated. They dilate arterioles by preventing the formation of angiotensin II, which causes arterioles to constrict and block the action of ACEs, which convert angiotensin I to angiotensin II.

Cough is a common side effect from this drug. In patients for whom an ACE inhibitor and diuretic combination are indicated but not tolerated, angiotensin-II receptor antagonist (e.g., losartan) and diuretic combinations may be used.

Beta-blockers
(Include acebutolol, atenolol, betaxolol, bisoprolol, carteolol, metoprolol, nadolol, penbutolol, pindolol, propranolol, and timolol)

This group of drugs acts by blocking the effects of the sympathetic division, the part of the nervous system that can rapidly respond to stress by increasing blood pressure. Side effects from beta blockers can include dizziness, fainting, bronchospasm, bradycardia, heart failure, possible masking of low blood sugar levels, impaired peripheral circulation, insomnia, fatigue, shortness of breath, depression, Raynaud's phenomenon,

(continued)

Box 3. I   Safe Use of Antihypertensive Medications (continued)

vivid dreams, hallucinations, sexual dysfunction, and, with some beta-blockers, an increased triglyceride level.

Calcium channel blockers
(Include amlodipine, diltiazem [sustained-release only], felodipine, isradipine, nicardipine, nifedipine [sustained-release only], nisoldipine, and verapamil)

The action of these drugs causes arterioles to dilate by a completely different mechanism. Side effects from these drugs include headache, dizziness, flushing, fluid retention, problems in the heart's electrical conduction system (including heart block), bradycardia, heart failure, enlarged gums, and constipation. ACE inhibitors and calcium channel blockers may be prescribed in combination to lower blood pressure, as may other combinations.

Alpha-blockers (doxazosin, prazosin, terazosin) *and angiotensin II blockers* (candesartan, eprosartan, irbesartan, losartan, telmisartan, valsartan) are among the other drugs that could be prescribed for hypertension management.

Diuretics
Diuretics are commonly used in combination with antihypertensive medications. They blunt the sodium- and water-retaining effects of many other antihypertensive drugs such as beta blockers, cause blood vessels to dilate, and help the kidneys eliminate salt and water, which reduces fluid volume throughout the body, thereby lowering blood pressure.

General considerations:
- Monitor patients closely when therapy is initiated. Some antihypertensives can initially cause significant hypotension. Advise patients to change positions slowly to prevent falls.
- If diuretics are prescribed, monitor for diuretic-induced dehydration.
- Ensure that patients obtain lab work as ordered. Monitoring of serum potassium is especially important when

(continued)

patients are receiving ACE inhibitors with potassium or potassium-sparing diuretics.
- Monitor patients for side effects.
- Reinforce to patients the importance of adhering to treatment even when symptoms are absent.
- Some antihypertensives should not be abruptly discontinued. Advise patients to check with their physicians before discontinuing these drugs.
- Be alert to interactions:
  - Antihypertensive drugs can increase the effects of barbiturates, insulin, oral antidiabetic drugs, sedatives, and thiazide diuretics.
  - The effects of antihypertensives can be decreased by amphetamines, antacids, antihistamines, salicylates, and tricyclic antidepressants.
  - Verapamil can increase the blood digoxin level.
  - The effects of propranolol can be increased by cimetidine, ciprofloxacin, diuretics.
  - Grapefruit juice can affect the bioavailability and alter the effects of calcium-channel blockers.
  - Individual drugs have specific interactions; carefully review the drug literature to learn about them.

═══════════════════════════ *FAST FACTS in a NUTSHELL*

At-home self-measurement can prove an effective means to monitor blood pressure, and has been endorsed by major groups such as the American Heart Association and the Preventive Cardiovascular Nurses Association (Pickering et al., 2008). The American Heart Association website (www.heart.org) has a page describing home blood pressure monitoring and can be a useful resource.

Coronary Artery Disease

Coronary artery disease (CAD), also called coronary heart disease, is a narrowing of the arteries that supply blood to the heart due to the build-up of plaque. The effects of the oxygen-deprived heart muscle can be angina or myocardial infarction. Over time, CAP can lead to HF and arrhythmias.

[**Clinical Snapshot**]

Mrs. E. experienced "white coat syndrome," in which her blood pressures rose when being examined by a health care professional. As a means to evaluate her normal blood pressure, she was instructed to monitor and record her blood pressure at home and bring the record to visits with her health care provider. Mrs. E. was instructed of the proper procedure for taking her blood pressure. She was also instructed not to independently stop taking her antihypertensive medication, even if her blood pressure readings were within a normal range, and that self-monitoring does not replace the need for regular visits to her health care provider.

Angina

Myocardial ischemia results in the pain of the anginal syndrome; however, in older adults the presentation of these symptoms can by atypical. Pain may be less severe and more diffuse than that which occurs in younger persons. There can be precardial pain radiating down the left arm as the condition progresses, along with syncope, coughing, confusion, and heavy perspiration.

FAST FACTS in a NUTSHELL

The patient experiencing angina may report a vague substernum discomfort, which often occurs after consuming a large meal, thereby sometimes causing it to be mistakenly attributed to indigestion.

Recurrent episodes of angina can lead to the development of small areas of myocardial necrosis and fibrosis. This weakens the heart and heightens the risk of HF. This reinforces the importance of effective prevention of anginal attacks.

Nitroglycerin is used to prevent and treat anginal attacks. Lower dosages may be prescribed for older adults due to the tendency of this drug to cause a reduction in blood pressure. To ensure the patient does not swallow the sublingual tablet, thereby interfering with its absorption, remind the patient about the placement of the tablet and instruct the patient to not swallow saliva for several minutes. Long-acting nitrates typically are not prescribed for older adults.

FAST FACTS in a NUTSHELL

The reduction in blood pressure that occurs after administration of a nitroglycerin tablet can cause dizziness and fainting, leading to a fall. To prevent injury, caution the patient to sit or lie down after taking the medication.

It is useful to help the patient identify factors (e.g., cold wind, emotional stress, strenuous activity) that trigger anginal attacks and develop strategies for avoiding or reducing them. As anemia, tachycardia, arrhythmias, and hyperthyroidism can increase the risk for angina, proper management of these conditions is integral to the care plan.

Myocardial Infarction

The incidence of myocardial infarction (MI) increases with age. Men with a history of hypertension and arteriosclerosis are at particularly high risk for MI.

MIs may not be identified in a timely manner in older persons due to an atypical presentation of symptoms. For example, pain can be absent, less severe, or present in the neck, back, or entire chest. Symptoms that could indicate MI include:

- Delirium
- Sense of tightness or pressure in chest
- Decreased blood pressure
- Dyspnea, shortness of breath
- Moist, pale skin
- Weakness
- Numbness in arms, neck, or back
- Nausea, vomiting
- Reduced urinary output (anuria can occur as MI progresses)

With any suspicion of an MI, the patient should be evaluated. Tests could include an ECG and angiogram; in some cases, cardiac catheterization can be performed. Sedimentation rate will be among the blood tests evaluated and with an MI will be elevated. Arrhythmias will be present, progressing to fibrillation and death if untreated. Vital signs should be monitored.

Support the treatment plan, which could include:

- Administration of oxygen to relieve hypoxic heart muscles. Older adults are at high risk for carbon dioxide retention; therefore, lower oxygen administration levels may be ordered and should be closely monitored. Blood gases are evaluated regularly.

FAST FACTS in a NUTSHELL

Older adults who have hypoxia may not display cyanosis, but instead demonstrate restlessness, irritability, and difficulty breathing.

- Administration of medications, including analgesics, nitroglycerin, antidysrhythmics, or digitalis. Thrombolytic therapy is often used and demands close nursing observation to detect signs of bleeding.
- Support of limbs. Note adverse reactions.
- Relief of pain and anxiety.
- Monitoring of intake and output, elimination pattern. Note anuria and straining due to constipation.
- Observation for complications such as congestive HF (evidenced through dyspnea, cough, rales, rhonchi) and shock (evidenced through decreased blood pressure; increased pulse; decreased urine output; restlessness; cool, moist skin). The physician should be made aware of any new or changed symptoms that are detected.

Extended periods of complete bedrest typically are not recommended. The patient will initially be able to sit in an armchair with arms supported to avoid strain on the heart, followed by ambulation within a few days of the MI (if there are no complications present). Early mobility post-MI not only offers cardiovascular benefits, but also helps to prevent the complications associated with immobility.

Hyperlipidemia

Age-related increases in LDL cholesterol and conditions prevalent in late life that cause lipoprotein disorders (e.g., uncontrolled diabetes, hypothyroidism, uremia) contribute to an increased prevalence of hyperlipidemia in the older population.

For diagnostic purposes, a full lipid profile rather than just a plasma total cholesterol level is recommended. Fasting 12 hours prior to testing is required for a definitive screening. HDL levels greater than 60 mg/dL and LDL levels less than 160 mg/dL are desirable.

FAST FACTS in a NUTSHELL

An HDL level greater than 60 mg/dL is desirable; triglycerides greater than 200 mg/dL are borderline and greater than 240 mg/dL are high.

An LDL less than 100 mg/dL is recommended for people with coronary heart disease or diabetes; a level less than 130 mg/dL is advised for persons without coronary heart disease or diabetes who have two or more coronary risk factors. LDL less than 160 mg/dL is desirable for persons without coronary heart disease or diabetes who have one or no risk factors.

When abnormal levels are found there should be an assessment of factors that could be responsible, such as a diet high in saturated fat or cholesterol; excessive alcohol intake; poorly controlled diabetes; or use of beta-blockers, corticosteroids, or estrogen. When none of these factors are present, there could be a familial lipoprotein disorder responsible.

Preferably, diet modifications and exercise are the initial approaches to treating hyperlipidemia. Nurses should reinforce good dietary practices, such as:

- Reducing the intake of egg yolks, whole milk, cream, red meat, and organ meat, and instead consuming skim milk, nonfat cottage cheese, fish, chicken, and turkey
- Increasing the intake of soluble fibers (e.g., oats, barley)
- Consuming plenty of fresh fruits and vegetables

Increasing exercise and maintaining weight within a normal range are positive lifestyle practices that assist in the management of this condition.

When dietary and lifestyle changes alone do not assist with returning levels to normal, medications may be prescribed. For elevated LDL cholesterol the drugs of first choice are the HMG CoA reductase inhibitors (e.g., atorvastatin, fluvastatin, lovastatin, pravastatin, rosuvastatin, and simvastatin). Statin drugs are very effective for lowering LDL cholesterol levels and have few immediate short-term side effects. Bile acid sequestrants (cholestyramine, colestipol), nicotinic acid (niacin [Nicolar]), 3-hydroxy-3-methylglutaryl-coenzyme, fibric acid derivatives (gemfibrozil, clofibrate), and omega-3 fatty acids (fish oils) can also be used.

Varicose Veins

The loss of vessel elasticity and strength that occurs with age, combined with a history of low exercise levels and occupations requiring considerable standing, cause varicosities to be a common finding among older adults. Varicosities will be detected upon physical examination by the presence of dilated, tortous veins, particularly in the lower extremities. The patient may report experiencing cramping and dull pain of the legs. Ulcers may be noted in the affected area due to the high susceptibility to trauma and infection; the risk for ulcerative lesions is especially high in people who are obese or who have diabetes. Persons with significant varicosities may get dizzy when rising from a lying position due to the localizations of blood in the lower extremity and consequent reduction of cerebral circulation.

A goal of treatment is to reduce venous stasis by promoting venous return. Measures to achieve this include:

- Elevating the legs periodically
- Walking and engaging in other exercise to enhance circulation
- Properly applying elastic stockings that may be prescribed
- Avoiding constricting clothing
- Not crossing legs while sitting or standing for prolonged periods
- Avoiding trauma to the legs
- Reporting new areas of discoloration and lesions to the health care provider

PROMOTING CARDIOVASCULAR HEALTH

The high prevalence of cardiovascular conditions in the older population and the impact of these conditions on the quality of life suggest that nurses should assist older persons in developing lifestyle practices that promote cardiovascular health. Nursing actions should include:

- Instructing on a diet that controls calories, fat, and sodium intake and encourages fiber, fish, poultry, nonfat dairy products, and fresh fruits and vegetables
- Encouraging exercise
- Instructing in stress management measures, such as relaxation exercises, meditation, and yoga
- Referring the patient to smoking cessation programs if he or she is a smoker
- Ensuring that the patient understands the dosage, administration, purpose, side effects, and adverse effects of all medications used
- Instructing the patient on signs and symptoms related to cardiovascular conditions and complications that should be reported to the physician

4

Respiratory System

Cigarette smoking, exposure to air pollution, and repeated infections are among the insults that can affect the health of the respiratory system for many adults in late life. These factors, combined with age-related changes and immobility associated with geriatric conditions, impact respiratory function and the prevalence of pulmonary disease. Pulmonary disease is a leading cause of disability and ranks as the fourth leading cause of death for people over 70 years of age. Because impaired respiratory function can result in activity limitations, respiratory infections, and a poor quality of life, nurses need to ensure older adults engage in actions to promote optimal respiratory function.

Objectives

In this chapter you will learn to:

1. Identify age-related changes to the respiratory system
2. Describe the process for assessing the respiratory system
3. Describe the symptoms and care of the older patient who has influenza

4. Describe the symptoms and care of the older patient who has pneumonia
5. Describe the symptoms and care of the older patient who has chronic obstructive pulmonary disease (COPD)
6. Outline the steps of providing postural drainage for older adults
7. Describe precautions in administering oxygen to older adults

AGE-RELATED CHANGES

The respiratory system experiences many changes with age that heighten the risk for infection and potentially interfere with normal activities. These changes include:

- Less supporting connective tissue in the nose, which can lead to nasal septum deviations that interfere with the passage of air
- Thicker mucus in the nasopharynx due to reduced submucosal gland secretions; there is more difficulty expelling mucus
- Rigidity of the trachea and rib cage due to calcification of cartilage
- Blunting of the laryngeal and coughing reflexes, leading to reduced coughing
- Reduction in size and weight of lungs
- Reduction in elastic collagen and elastin in lungs, causing less elastic recoil during expiration
- Greater use of accessory muscles during expiration
- Fewer functional capillaries, development of fibrous tissue, and less elasticity of alveoli
- Increase in anterior-posterior chest diameter

These changes result in reduced lung expansion during respiration, poor inflation of the base of the lungs, and more difficulty expelling foreign or accumulated matter from the lungs. Less effective exhalation leads to increased residual volume, which causes reduced vital capacity and breathing capacity. Even in the absence of significant respiratory disease, there can be dyspnea when extra demands increase respirations, as can occur during exercise. In addition, the risk for developing respiratory infections is high.

The effects of aging on other bodily systems can affect the health of the respiratory system as well. A slight kyphosis can occur due to a loss of skeletal strength in the thorax and diaphragm, reducing full lung expansion. Drier mucous membrane associated with reduced bodily fluids makes it more difficult to remove secretions from the lungs. A weaker gag reflex, slower gastric motility, and relaxation of sphincters increase the risk for aspiration of food into the lungs. Not only do common aging changes external to the respiratory system increase the risk of infections, but they can also interfere with early detection. For example, altered pain sensations and lower normal body temperatures can delay the detection of a respiratory infection.

FAST FACTS in a NUTSHELL

Cigarette smoking can compound the effects of aging on the respiratory system and heighten the risk for respiratory infection and disease. Although the soundest practice for respiratory health is to not have a history of smoking, smoking cessation can benefit older adults who still engage in the practice.

ASSESSMENT CONSIDERATIONS

Often the presence of respiratory problems can be detected upon first contact with the patient by observing energy level; coloring; and the presence of dyspnea, abnormal respiratory rate or depth, coughing, or breath sounds.

Review the patient's history for known respiratory conditions, smoking history, and exposure to occupational pollutants. Question the patient about symptoms such as:

- Dyspnea
- Shortness of breath
- Coughing
- Expectoration of mucus
- Bloody mucus
- Chest pain or tightness
- Runny nose
- Wheezing

If symptoms are present, ask about frequency, characteristics, and factors that trigger them.

Expose the chest for inspection:

- Look for equal expansion of both sides during respirations, scars, discoloration, structural abnormalities.
- There may be some barreling of the chest as a result of aging, but the anterior-posterior chest diameter normally should not be greater than the lateral diameter.
- A ruddy complexion of the face, neck, and chest can be associated with emphysema; a bluish-gray coloring can occur with chronic bronchitis.

Auscultate the lungs:

- Close the door to the room and turn off televisions and radios to create as quiet an environment as possible.
- Assist the patient in sitting upright.
- Rub the diaphragm of the stethoscope to warm it prior to placing it on the patient's bare chest.

═══════════════ *FAST FACTS in a NUTSHELL*

To accurately hear breath sounds, do not listen through the patient's clothing; place the stethoscope directly on the patient's chest. Be alert to the fact that rubbing the stethoscope in the area of chest hair can create sounds that can be confused with abnormal breath sounds.

- Begin at the base of the lungs and work up the back. Listen for at least two full respirations.

  Determine if the sounds are clear and normal, or abnormal. Breath sounds can be reduced with emphysema, pleural effusion, or conditions causing shallow respiration. Abnormal breath sounds include:

- *Rales* or *crackles:* a crackling sound heard at the end of inspiration, indicating extra interstitial fluid
- *Rhonchi:* a rattling sound heard at the end of expiration, indicating increased mucus production and partial airway obstruction
- *Wheezes:* a groaning sound, indicating the presence of large amounts of mucus

Proceed with palpation of the chest for tactile fremitus (vibratory tremors):

- Using the ulnar surface of the hands, place hands on both sides of the chest at the top area of the lungs, and ask the patient to say "99."
- Move hands down along other areas of the lungs and repeat.
- Fremitus is normally best felt in the upper lobes. Reduced fremitus in the upper lobes can be associated with COPD or pneumothorax; increased fremitus in the lower lobe can occur with pneumonia or a mass.

Percuss the lungs over the intercostal spaces from the top of the lungs to the bases, comparing sides. To percuss:

- Place the middle finger of your nondominant hand firmly on the chest, over an intercostal space
- Using the middle finger of the opposite hand, tap over the distal interphalangeal joint of the finger that is on the chest several times (the tapping motion should come from the wrist, not the movement of the whole arm)
- Note the sound produced
- Repeat for the opposite side

Normally, percussion of the lung field reveals a clear, low-pitched sound known as *resonance*. A *dull* sound indicates the filling of a space, as in consolidation or pleural effusion. *Hyperresonance,* a high-pitched, drum-like sound, can reveal an overinflated organ, as may occur with COPD.

FAST FACTS in a NUTSHELL

The high prevalence of health conditions in older adults makes them likely to be using medications that can mask symptoms of respiratory infections. This reinforces the importance of obtaining a complete listing of all prescription and over-the-counter medications used and in performing a complete assessment of the respiratory system, even if symptoms are not apparent.

CONDITIONS

Influenza

Influenza is a significant threat to older adults, who account for most of the deaths from this infection. A major reason for this is due to age-related changes that reduce respiratory activity and impair the immune response to the virus. Symptoms include aching muscles, fever (although it can be at lower levels than what occurs in persons of younger ages), sore throat, and nonproductive cough.

FAST FACTS in a NUTSHELL

Older adults with chronic cardiac, respiratory, or metabolic disease are at high risk for developing bacterial pneumonia when they experience influenza.

Due to their high risk for contracting an influenza infection and developing complications when they do, active measures to prevent this infection are essential.

FAST FACTS in a NUTSHELL

All persons over age 65 should receive the influenza vaccine; exceptions would be persons with febrile conditions, egg allergy, and a history of Guillain-Barré syndrome. Although older persons typically have lower antibody titers after vaccination than younger adults, vaccination can prevent severe complications associated with influenza, even if it does not prevent the infection itself. Because influenza is acquired through inhalation of infected droplets, it is important to urge patients to avoid contact with persons with known or suspected influenza. Because immunity gradually declines, annual re-vaccination is necessary.

It is important to monitor the blood levels of carbamazepine, phenobarbital, phenytoin, theophylline, and warfarin in persons using these drugs who are vaccinated, and observe for toxic reactions, as drug levels can rise to toxic levels within 1 to 4 weeks after vaccination.

Older adults who develop influenza need to be closely monitored and encouraged to consume adequate liquids and engage in deep breathing exercises throughout the day to avoid complications. Secondary bacterial pneumonia is the primary risk, with nonpulmonary complications being a temporary loss of smell or taste, myositis, pericarditis, Guillain-Barré syndrome, and encephalitis.

Pneumonia

Pneumonia is a major risk to older adults and one of the leading causes of death for this population. A variety of factors contribute to the high incidence of pneumonia in older adults, including:

- Lower resistance to infection
- Higher incidence of conditions that reduce mobility
- Reduced chest expansion
- Greater risk of aspiration of foreign matter into the lungs due to decreased sensitivity of pharyngeal reflexes
- Increased prevalence of respiratory conditions that produce mucus and create bronchial obstruction
- Greater risk of being in hospitals or nursing homes and developing nosocomial pneumonia

In addition to having a higher risk for developing pneumonia, older adults may have delayed diagnosis of this infection due to altered presentation of symptoms:

- Lower normal body temperatures can cause fever to be present at lower levels than would be expected for younger persons.
- Pleuritic pain may be less severe than what younger individuals experience.
- Symptoms could include fatigue; a slight cough; and rapid, shallow respirations. Cerebral hypoxia can cause confusion and restlessness.

The care of older adults with pneumonia is similar to that of other age groups. Due to the altered presentation of symptoms, changes in status can be missed; therefore, close observation and monitoring are needed.

FAST FACTS in a NUTSHELL

The Centers for Disease Control and Prevention (CDC) recommends a pneumococcal vaccination and a one-time booster after 5 years if the person was under age 65 years when the initial vaccination was administered. When this vaccination is administered, document the administration of the vaccine, along with the name of the manufacturer, lot number, and expiration date. The CDC also advises that if there is doubt whether the vaccine has already been given, it is best to administer the vaccine rather than risk pneumonia.

Chronic Obstructive Pulmonary Disease (COPD)

COPD encompasses a group of diseases that include a form of asthma, chronic bronchitis, and emphysema. They are grouped together due to the airflow obstruction that they each produce. The incidence of COPD is higher in smokers and women.

Asthma

Asthma can be a lifelong condition or one that has developed in late life. Symptoms are similar to that which occurs in other age groups; however, older adults with asthma risk complications such as bronchiectasis and cardiac problems due to the stress exerted on the heart. Older adults also have a higher mortality from asthma.

FAST FACTS in a NUTSHELL

Even if patients have had a long history of asthma, it can be useful to review factors that precipitate attacks.

In addition to reviewing asthma triggers with the patient, it is beneficial to assess the patient's use of aerosol nebulizers. Difficulty using the nebulizer interferes with the inhalant medication adequately penetrating the lungs. If this proves to be a problem,

[Clinical Snapshot]

Ms. J. has had asthma throughout her adult life. She has identified certain allergens, such as sawdust, that trigger her asthma attacks; however, she has not fully understood that her emotions contribute to her attacks as well. By reviewing what precipitated her most recent attacks, the nurse was able to aid Ms. J. in identifying emotional triggers and developing strategies to manage her reactions differently to avoid triggering future attacks.

consult with the pharmacist about special devices (e.g., spacers, holding chambers) that may be helpful for the specific problem. If a sympathomimetic bronchodilating nebulizer is used, review the frequency of use, as overuse risks having the patient develop cardiac arrhythmias and cardiac arrest. Consult with the physician about the use of steroid inhalants that have a lower risk of systemic absorption and adverse reactions than the older steroids.

Chronic Bronchitis

Chronic bronchitis results from recurrent inflammation and mucus production in the bronchial tubes, which, over time, produce blockage and scarring that restrict airflow. Symptoms often develop gradually and include:

- Persistent, productive cough
- Wheezing
- Shortness of breath
- Recurrent respiratory infections
- Difficulty breathing in cold, damp weather due to bronchospasm

Emphysema may develop with time.

Treatment priorities include removing secretions and preventing airway obstruction. Older patients need to be reminded to consume adequate fluids and expectorate secretions.

Emphysema

A variety of factors contribute to the high incidence of emphysema in older adults, including:

- Morphologic changes in the lungs, which include distention of the alveolar sacs, rupture of the alveolar walls, and destruction of the alveolar capillary bed
- Chronic bronchitis
- Chronic irritation from dusts or certain air pollutants
- Cigarette smoking

Symptoms occur gradually and include:

- Increased dyspnea that is not relieved by sitting upright, as it may have been in the past
- Chronic cough
- Significant effort required for breathing
- Recurrent respiratory infections
- Fatigue, weakness
- Anorexia, weight loss, malnutrition

Complications can develop, such as congestive heart failure and cardiac arrhythmias.

Treatment typically consists of postural drainage (Box 4.1), bronchodilators, the avoidance of stressful situations, and breathing exercises.

The older patient may have insufficient energy to consume adequate food and fluid; nurses need to assess for this and arrange for dietary interventions that can facilitate intake (e.g., frequent small feedings and high-protein supplements).

The age-related changes that are experienced in the respiratory system result in less effective exhalation and increased residual volume. Emphysema heightens the effects of these changes and increases the carbon dioxide that remains in the lungs. For this reason, if oxygen is ordered for older patients with emphysema, extreme caution is needed due to their high risk for carbon dioxide narcosis. Attention to keeping the oxygen level at that which is prescribed is important. Individuals unaware of the dynamics of carbon dioxide

Box 4.1 Postural Drainage in Older Adults

Postural drainage can be prescribed for removing bronchial secretions. Although the basic procedure is the same as with other adults, some slight adjustments to the procedure are done when performing postural drainage on older adults:

- If aerosol medications are prescribed, administer them first.
- Select the position for postural drainage based on the individual patient and the portion of the lung involved.
- The older patient needs to change positions slowly and be allowed a few minutes to rest between position changes to adjust to the new position.
- The usual last position for postural drainage—lying face down across the bed with the head at floor level—may be stressful for the older person and have adverse effects. Ask the physician if this position should be included.
- Use gentle motions, as the older patient's tissues and bones are more fragile and injure more easily.
- Discontinue the procedure immediately if dyspnea, palpitation, chest pain, diaphoresis, apprehension, or any other sign of distress occurs.
- Provide oral hygiene and a period of rest after performing the procedure.
- Document the patient's tolerance of the procedure and the amount and characteristic of the mucus drained.

accumulation in older lungs may see the older patient having difficulty breathing and adjust the gauge to a higher infusion level; this results in higher levels of carbon dioxide developing, leading to carbon dioxide narcosis. All caregivers need to understand this and ensure the prescribed level is maintained. (See Box 4.2, Safe Use of Oxygen in Older Adults.)

Box 4.2   Safe Use of Oxygen With Older Adults

- Evaluate and recommend the method of administration that will be most effective for the individual patient. Nasal cannulas may not be effective for older patients who breathe by mouth or have poor control in keeping their lips sealed most of the time. Emaciated patients whose facial structures do not allow for a tight seal of a face mask may lose a significant portion of oxygen through leakage. Patients with anxiety or behavioral problems can resist being inside an oxygen tent and will not gain full therapeutic benefit
- Check the gauge frequently to ensure that it is set at the prescribed level
- Check the oxygen flow for any interruption or blockage from an empty tank, kinked tubing, or other problems
- Ensure the patient's nasal passages are regularly cleaned to maintain patency
- Note indications of insufficient oxygenation; some older persons will not become cyanotic when hypoxic
- Observe for symptoms of carbon dioxide narcosis, which include confusion, muscle twitching, visual defects, profuse perspiration, hypotension, progressive degrees of circulatory failure, and cerebral depression, which may be displayed as increased sleeping or a deep comatose state
- Ensure blood gases are monitored

In addition, for patients using oxygen at home:

- Assess the patient's knowledge of safe oxygen use and precautions; provide education to address deficits
- Ensure the home environment is assessed for safety and precautions are explained (e.g., not using oxygen in the kitchen where there is a stove with flames)
- Ensure regular contact and monitoring through a home health agency has been arranged and occurs
- Reinforce that the oxygen needs to be kept at the prescribed level

FAST FACTS in a NUTSHELL

A challenge for the patient with COPD is breathing adequately enough to expel carbon dioxide and secretions from the lungs. Abdominal breathing exercises can assist with expirations and movement of secretions.

[Clinical Snapshot]

Seventy-five year-old Mr. W has COPD as a result of decades of cigarette smoking and needs to learn abdominal breathing exercises. The nurse begins teaching Mr. W the exercises by having him hold a pillow against his abdomen and instructing him to take a deep inspiration to the count of five as he pushes the pillow out with his abdomen. The nurse then asks him to lean forward, exhale with pursed lips to the count of ten, and pull in his abdomen as he pushes the pillow toward his abdomen. During this process the nurse encourages Mr. W to cough and expel any loosened secretions. Mr. W is advised to do several sets of these exercises at various times throughout the day. Having learned that he watches news on the television several times throughout the day, the nurse suggests that as a memory aid Mr. W do the exercises whenever he watches the news.

Lung Cancer

Lung cancer rates are highest in the older population, with men and Black individuals having the highest incidence and mortality rates. Chronic exposure to cigarette smoke, asbestos, coal gas, radon gas, and air pollutants contribute to the development of lung cancer, which reinforces the importance of obtaining smoking and occupational history during the assessment. Symptoms, which may not be present in the early stage of the disease, include:

- Dyspnea
- Coughing
- Chest pain

- Fatigue
- Anorexia
- Wheezing
- Recurrent upper respiratory infections

Chest roentgenogram, sputum cytology, bronchoscopy, and biopsy confirm the diagnosis. The principles of treatment are similar for persons of any age and include surgery, chemotherapy, or radiotherapy. Other conditions that the older patient may have can affect treatment choices and prognosis.

5

Gastrointestinal System

The healthy consumption and digestion of food and elimination of wastes remain essential in late life; however, age-related changes and health conditions to which older adults are more susceptible challenge these functions. Interventions to compensate for changes to the gastrointestinal (GI) system, identify disorders early, and ensure adequate treatment of conditions affecting this system contribute to a positive nutritional state and overall health for older individuals.

Objectives

In this chapter you will learn to:

1. Identify age-related changes to the GI system
2. Describe components of the assessment of the GI system
3. Recognize the clinical signs and describe the care of older patients with:
   - Anorexia
   - Dry mouth (xerostomia)
   - Oral disease
   - Dysphagia
   - Hiatal hernia

- Dehydration
- Constipation
- Fecal impaction
- Hemorrhoids
- Diverticular disease
- Colorectal cancer

AGE-RELATED CHANGES

Virtually all parts of the GI system are affected by the aging process and although these changes may not be life-threatening, they often tend to be changes that affect daily life. Changes to the GI system include:

- Harder and more brittle tooth enamel; reduced production of dentin (the layer beneath the enamel); shrinkage and fibrosis of root pulp; retraction of gingiva

FAST FACTS in a NUTSHELL

Tooth loss does not normally occur with age; however, a history of poor dental care, dietary factors, and the ease at which teeth fracture in late life contribute to a high prevalence of tooth loss among older adults. Fortunately, improved diets and dental care will enable greater numbers of people to enter their senior years with improved dental status.

- Less acute taste sensations, particularly affecting sweet sensations located on the tip of the tongue
- Sublingual varicosities; loss of papillae on the tongue
- Reduced saliva production; reduction in salivary ptyalin affecting the breakdown of starches; increased incidence of xerostomia (dry mouth)
- Decreased tongue pressure and muscle strength, which can interfere with mastication and swallowing
- Development of presbyesophagus, a condition characterized by decreased intensity of propulsive waves and increased frequency of nonpropulsive waves in the esophagus, which

slows esophageal motility; slower esophageal emptying, which heightens risk for aspiration
- Reduced gastric secretion of hydrochloric acid and pepsin; atrophy of gastric mucosa
- Decreased cells on the absorbing surface of intestinal walls; slower fat absorption; more difficulty absorbing dextrose, xylose, calcium, iron, and vitamins B, B12, and D
- Reduced awareness of need to evacuate due to slower transmission of neural impulses to the lower bowel
- Increased incidence of gallstones due to decreased bile salt synthesis and less efficient cholesterol stabilization and absorption
- Dilation and distension of pancreatic ducts

These changes can interfere with a healthy nutritional intake. To avoid this problem and compensate for the effects of age-related changes, actions can be taken such as:

- Practicing good oral hygiene
- Obtaining regular dental care
- Ingesting adequate fluids
- Eating in an upright position and remaining upright for at least 20 minutes after meals
- Including fiber-rich foods in the diet
- Establishing a regular time for bowel elimination

ASSESSMENT CONSIDERATIONS

The techniques of interview, inspection, auscultation, percussion, and palpation are used in the assessment of the GI system. Because symptoms of disturbances in the GI system typically are quite noticeable to the patient (e.g., nausea, indigestion, diarrhea, cramping), the patient often can identify problem areas that require special focus.

Upon first contact with the patient, some clues of GI problems can be detected, such as:

- *Apparent weakness:* This can be associated with malnutrition, fluid and electrolyte imbalances, or GI bleeding.
- *Body size:* Both emaciation and obesity signal problems that require further exploration.

- *Pallor:* GI bleeding can lead to an anemic state.
- *Skin dryness, rashes, itching, or discoloration:* Nutritional deficiencies, allergies, and liver disorders can cause skin issues.

In some situations, the patient may not independently contribute certain GI symptoms or changes, believing they are to be expected with aging (e.g., tooth loss, indigestion, weight changes), so it is beneficial to ask specific questions; these could include:

- How do you care for your teeth or dentures, if they are present? When was the last time you visited a dentist? Do you have any pain, bleeding, sores, or other problems with your gums or mouth?
- Do you have any problems tasting the flavor of foods? If so, what do you do to compensate for that (e.g., add salt, sugar)?
- Have you noticed any changes in your appetite?
- Have you been experiencing nausea, vomiting, indigestion, diarrhea, constipation, gas, or bloody or discolored stools? Do you have stomach, intestinal, or rectal pain?
- What is your typical diet?
- How often do you have a bowel movement? Do you have to use a laxative, suppository, or enema? If so, how often?
- Have you had a colonoscopy? When was that and what were the results?

Explore responses that could indicate symptoms or possible deviations from normal.

A useful approach to the physical examination is to assess from the entrance of the system to its end, reviewing:

- *Lips:* Note color, moisture, and symmetry. Insufficient oxygen can cause a bluish discoloration to the lips. Dryness can indicate dehydration. Note lesions or sores and ask the patient about the length of time they have been present. Fissures and cracks can result from riboflavin deficiencies or overclosure of the mouth due to missing teeth or poor-fitting dentures.
- *Oral cavity:* Examine the mouth using a tongue depressor and flashlight. The mucosa normally should appear moist and pink; a pigmented oral mucosa can be a normal finding in dark-skinned individuals. Although older adults may have

a drier oral mucosa than younger persons, extreme dryness could indicate dehydration. White patches that appear like beads of dried milk can be associated with moniliasis (thrush) infections. Note discoloration, inflammation, and bleeding of the gums. Periodontal disease, the primary cause of tooth loss in older adults, is characterized by redness, swelling, and bleeding of the gums. Dilantin therapy and leukemia can also cause swelling of the gums. The top and bottom surfaces of the tongue should be inspected. A coated tongue is often the result of poor oral hygiene or low fluid intake; wiping the tongue with gauze can aid in removing accumulated materials and obtaining a truer assessment. A smooth, red tongue can indicate a deficiency of iron, niacin, or vitamin B12. Varicosities are not uncommon on the undersurface of the older adult's tongue. As cancerous lesions are more common on the undersurface of the tongue, it is important to inspect this area carefully. The patient should be able to move the tongue from side to side and up and down. Note unusual odors when examining the mouth, which can occur with poor oral hygiene, oral cavity disease, lung abcesses, and some systemic conditions.

- *Pharynx:* Test the function of the vagus nerve (which causes the soft palate to rise and block the nasopharynx during swallowing, thereby preventing aspiration). Press a tongue depressor on the middle portion of the tongue and ask the patient to say "ah." Normally, the soft palate will rise when the patient says "ah"; if it does not rise properly, the patient could be at risk of aspiration of food. Ask about swallowing problems and soreness. Redness and white patches in the throat usually are associated with infection; if present, obtain a culture.

- *Abdomen:* All methods of examination—inspection, auscultation, palpation, and percussion—are used in the assessment of the abdomen. To prepare for the examination, offer the patient the opportunity to void and position him or her in a comfortable, supine position. Findings should be described based on the quadrant of the abdomen where they are found; the umbilicus is at the center of the abdomen and is the point where the horizontal and vertical lines dividing the abdomen intersect. Inspect the abdomen, noting general skin color and condition, rashes, scars, striae (stretch marks, which are pink or blue if recently developed and become silvery white with time), bulging, distension, and asymmetry. The abdomen should rise and fall in harmony with respirations. Hernias can be identified by having the patient lift the head while in the supine position.

FAST FACTS in a NUTSHELL

A stethoscope is used to assess the abdomen. Intestinal sounds are high-pitched and best heard using the diaphragm of the stethoscope. Vascular sounds are heard holding the bell portion of the stethoscope lightly against the abdomen over areas of major arteries. Exerting too much pressure on the stethoscope can cause sounds to be missed.

Auscultate all four quadrants, listening for bowel sounds, which can occur irregularly, once every 5 to 15 seconds. If no bowel sounds are heard after listening for a few minutes, try to trigger activity by flicking your finger on the abdominal wall. Murmurs over major vessels can indicate dilated or constricted vessels.

Percussing the abdomen can aid in identifying fluid, gas, and masses. Dullness indicates a solid mass; tympany indicates the presence of gas.

Palpation is beneficial in identifying abdominal abnormalities. Begin by using light palpation to determine the presence of tenderness, muscle resistance, and large masses.

FAST FACTS in a NUTSHELL

For light palpation, depress the pads, not the tips, of the fingers into the abdominal wall approximately 1 cm. Palpate all quadrants, noting areas of sensitivity, spasm, or rigidity. Follow this with moderate palpation of the quadrants using the side of the hand.

Masses should be described as to their location, size, shape, tenderness, and relation to activity (e.g., coughing, respiration). Some tenderness over the cecum, sigmoid colon, and aorta is normal. Tenderness can be associated with peritoneal irritation; if present, test for rebound tenderness by pushing the pads of the fingers deeply into the tender area and quickly withdrawing them.

- *Rectum:* The left lateral and standing positions are the most commonly used for rectal examination. In the standing position the patient flexes his or her hips to allow the upper extremity to rest across the examining table or bed. In the left lateral position, the patient rests on the left side, flexing the right hip and knee. Begin the examination by spreading the buttocks and inspecting the perianal region, noting external hemorrhoids, rashes, lesions, tumors, fissures, inflammation, or other unusual findings. By asking the patient to strain and bear down as though having a bowel movement, hemorrhoids and rectal prolapse can be revealed. As the patient bears down, gently insert a lubricated gloved finger into the anal canal toward the direction of the umbilicus, and palpate the rectal wall and canal by rotating the finger. Be alert to masses and other irregularities.

=== *FAST FACTS in a NUTSHELL*

A hard mass that blocks palpation during digital examination of the rectum could be a fecal impaction.

[Clinical Snapshot]

A caregiver has reported to the home health nurse that 80-year-old Mr. V is complaining of abdominal discomfort and has something that looks like diarrhea on his underpants. In examining Mr. V the nurse finds his abdomen to be distended and learns that he has not had a normal bowel movement for at least 4 days. As her agency permits her to do so, the nurse performs a rectal examination and feels a hard, moveable mass. Some oozing of diarrhea-like discharge is noted and fecal material is present on the nurse's withdrawn gloved finger, consistent with the findings of a fecal impaction.

The strength of the sphincter muscle can be assessed by asking the patient to tighten the muscles around the finger.

Upon withdrawal of the finger, examine the fecal matter that has adhered to the glove's surface for unusual color or content. Tarry black stool can be associated with upper GI bleeding; bright red stool can occur with lower bowel problems. Obstructive jaundice can cause the stool to lack pigmentation and appear gray or tan. Mucus particles can indicate an inflammatory process.

CONDITIONS

Anorexia

Loss of appetite is such a common problem among older adults that some believe it to be a natural part of aging. Although reductions in the senses of smell and taste, slower metabolism, and less energy expenditure contribute to a decreased appetite, there are other conditions that could contribute to anorexia that could be improved or that need to be evaluated, such as:

- Depression and other psychiatric disorders (studies have found that psychiatric disorders were present in most older adults with anorexia, with depression being the most common condition; Lapid et al., 2010)
- Poor dental status
- Digestive disorders
- Pain that limits ability to prepare or consume foods
- Fatigue
- Medication side effects
- Limited finances
- Hormonal deficiencies
- Undiagnosed diseases (e.g., cancer, chronic obstructive pulmonary disease)

Signs of anorexia could be reflected through:

- Weight loss
- Fatigue, weakness
- Disinterest in food
- Low food intake
- Altered mental status

FAST FACTS in a NUTSHELL

Sometimes the most obvious factor may not be the primary one responsible for anorexia.

[Clinical Snapshot]

Mrs. L, a new widow, was thought to have anorexia related to depression over the loss of her husband. In discussing and assessing the situation with Mrs. L, the nurse learns that without having her spouse to drive her to the supermarket and with the significant reduction in income experienced, Mrs. L is unable to afford a proper diet and has not wanted to burden others by admitting this. The nurse involved the social worker, who assisted Mrs. L in obtaining financial aid and arranging transportation to shop for food. These interventions improved her food intake.

Factors contributing to anorexia need to be explored and interventions to address them planned. Eating several smaller meals rather than a few large ones could improve intake. The physician and nutritionist should be consulted regarding the benefits of vitamin and mineral supplements and appetite stimulants.

Dry Mouth (Xerostomia)

In addition to a slight decline in saliva production with age, there are other factors that contribute to a dry mouth in late life, such as medications, mouth breathing, altered cognition, and Sjögren's syndrome, a disease of the immune system.

FAST FACTS in a NUTSHELL

Many of the medications used to treat geriatric conditions can cause dryness of the oral cavity. Among them are angiotensin-converting enzyme (ACE) inhibitors, anticholinergics, anticonvulsants, antidepressants, antihistamines, and antiparkinsonian drugs.

Frequent oral hygiene not only assists in moistening the mouth, but also in reducing the risk of dental disease that can arise from having insufficient saliva. Many patients are aided by sipping water and using sugar-free hard candies. Saliva substitutes are available if these measures are insufficient.

Oral Disease

Oral health contributes to a good nutritional intake, positive self-concept, and comfort; therefore it is important to promote dental care and oral health in late life. Regular brushing of teeth, gums, and the tongue, as well as flossing, are necessary measures. If dentures are worn, gentle gum massage with a toothbrush should be done. Regular visits to the dentist remain important.

FAST FACTS in a NUTSHELL

Regular visits to the dentist are important for older adults. Poor condition of the teeth can affect appetite, comfort, and socialization. Systemic infections can develop from untreated periodontal disease. Further, the presence of dentures doesn't eliminate the need for dental examination as changes in tissue structure can cause dentures to fit less well with time; in addition, the dentist can detect problems like oral cancers, which rise in incidence with age.

The teeth often show the effects of aging, evidenced by:

- Worn down surfaces
- Reduction in tooth enamel
- Varying degrees of root absorption
- Reduction in size and volume of pulp
- Increased tooth brittleness

The patient should be asked about dental care and the frequency of visits to the dentist. Misconceptions that dental visits are not necessary in late life need to be corrected. If expense is a problem, help the patient locate a free or inexpensive source of dental care.

Dysphagia

Dysphagia, difficulty swallowing, is estimated to affect approximately 20% of the population, with the highest prevalence among older adults (Keller, 2011). Among the most common causes are gastroesophageal reflux disease (GERD), stroke, structural disorders, and conditions that cause excessive coughing while eating or drinking.

FAST FACTS in a NUTSHELL

Dysphagia can be oropharyngeal or esophageal. Neurologic damage often causes oropharyngeal dysphagia, in which there is difficulty transferring food bolus or liquid from the mouth into the pharynx and esophagus. Esophageal dysphagia is characterized by difficulty with the transfer of food down the esophagus and is more common in persons with motility disorders, sphincter abnormalities, or mechanical obstructions caused by strictures.

It is estimated that only half of the people affected with dysphagia discuss the problem with their medical provider (Keller, 2011). As dysphagia increases the risk for aspiration and its serious consequences, asking about this problem while assessing older patients could prove useful. Questions that could aid in revealing dysphagia include:

- Do you cough or choke when eating or drinking?
- Does it sometimes feel like food is stuck in your throat?
- Does it ever feel that you are not swallowing food normally?
- Do you have difficulty swallowing certain foods?

A positive response warrants further evaluation. If the patient contributes that he or she has difficulty swallowing, ask:

- How long has this problem been present?
- How often does it happen?

- Are there other symptoms that occur with it, such as coughing, pain, or indigestion?
- Are there certain foods or forms of food (liquids, meats) that seem to cause this more than others?
- Is there anything you do that seems to help you swallow easier?
- Have you noticed any weight loss?

A modified barium swallow typically is ordered for patients with dysphagia. The cause of the problem (e.g., neurological disorder, mass) will determine the treatment. Speech therapists are often involved in recommending specific interventions, which could include patients' positions for eating and drinking, exercises to strengthen the muscles involved in swallowing, and techniques for safe eating and swallowing. Dieticians can suggest diet modifications that could prove beneficial, such as adding thickeners to liquids to facilitate swallowing. Caution is needed due to the high risk for aspiration.

Hiatal Hernia

The increased incidence of hiatal hernia with age results in nearly half of the people over age 50 experiencing this problem.

FAST FACTS in a NUTSHELL

There are two types of hiatal hernia: sliding (axial) and rolling (paraesophageal). The sliding type occurs when a part of the stomach and the junction of the stomach and esophagus slide through the diaphragm; this is the most common type. In the rolling type, the fundus and greater curvatures of the stomach roll up through the diaphragm.

Symptoms, which can be more pronounced when the patient is in a recumbent position, include:

- Heartburn (at times mistaken for cardiac pain)
- Dysphagia

- Belching
- Regurgitation, vomiting

Barium swallow and esophagoscopy are done to confirm the diagnosis. Medical management suffices for most patients and consists of:

- Weight reduction (if the patient is obese)
- Bland diet; reduced consumption of caffeinated and carbonated beverages, alcohol, and spicy foods
- Consuming several small-portioned meals rather than three large ones
- Not eating several hours prior to bedtime
- Milk or antacids for symptomatic relief
- Medications: H2 blockers (e.g., cimetidine, nizatidine, ranitidine), proton-pump inhibitors (lansoprazole, omeprazole)

Dehydration

Adequate hydration is an essential component of health, but one that becomes more challenging in late life due to age-related factors such as reduced sense of thirst, decreased intracellular fluid, decrease in fluid-rich muscle tissue, and less efficient renal handling of water and sodium. These factors heighten the risk for dehydration when factors are present that reduce fluid intake or cause excess fluid loss, such as:

- Vomiting
- Diarrhea
- Polyuria
- Profuse perspiration
- Medications (e.g., diuretics, laxatives)
- Altered mental status leading to insufficient intake
- Physical inability to consume fluids
- Self-imposed low fluid intake to reduce incontinence or need for toileting

These are not unusual situations in older persons due to the conditions that are highly prevalent in this population; therefore, signs of dehydration need to be regularly assessed. Signs of dehydration include:

- Dry oral mucosa and tongue
- Reduced saliva
- Decreased urine output
- Sunken eyes
- Weakness
- Tachycardia
- Increased body temperature
- Reduced urinary output; dark-colored urine
- Delirium

FAST FACTS in a NUTSHELL

Reduced skin elasticity with age causes skin turgor to be an unreliable indicator of dehydration in older patients.

Laboratory tests indicating dehydration include:

- BUN/creatinine ratio >25
- Serum sodium >150 mEq/L
- Serum osmolality >300 mmol/kg
- Urine specific gravity >1.029
- Urine osmolality >1050 mmol/kg

Addressing the underlying cause of the dehydration and restoring fluid balance must be done immediately to correct this life-threatening problem. Interventions can consist of intravenous fluid replacement, encouraging a specific volume of oral fluid intake, administering medications to treat an infection or stop diarrhea, or discontinuing diuretic therapy. Nurses assist by:

- Supporting the prescribed treatment
- Strictly monitoring intake and output
- Assessing vital signs and mental status every 4 hours or as ordered
- Weighing the patient daily and comparing current to previous weight

- Checking the skin status regularly; providing good skin care
- Developing a plan to address the patient's specific risks for dehydration and providing measures to eliminate or reduce those risks

Constipation

Constipation, the infrequent bowel elimination with the passage of passage of hard, dry feces or stool that is difficult to expel, is one of the most common conditions present in older adults. Factors contributing to constipation include:

- Slower peristalsis
- Inactivity, immobility
- Inadequate intake of bulk, fiber, or fluids
- Poor bowel habits (e.g., not establishing regular time for elimination, ignoring urge to defecate)
- Medications (e.g., iron, analgesics, sedatives, antipsychotics)
- Laxative abuse
- Pathologic conditions (e.g., hypothyroidism, hypercalcemia, dementia)

  Clinical signs of constipation include:

- Difficult passage of hard, dry stools
- Decreased frequency of bowel movements
- Abdominal fullness, discomfort, or distension
- Rectal fullness or pressure
- Flatulence
- Presence of hard stools in rectum felt during palpation
- Nausea, vomiting, anorexia
- Decreased activity

  In addition to the clinical signs, nurses should consider the following as part of the assessment:

- Bowel elimination history
- Character and frequency of stools

- Diet
- Prescription and over-the-counter medications used
- Supplements used
- Related signs and symptoms: rectal pain, low back pain, alternating constipation and diarrhea
- Auscultation of bowel sounds
- Palpation of abdomen and rectum

Identifying and correcting the factors that contribute to the constipation are important first steps. The following are additional interventions that could prove beneficial:

- Unless contraindicated, increase intake of foods that could promote bowel elimination, such as bran, whole grains, raw vegetables, prunes, spinach.
- Ask the patient to identify foods that have produced bowel movements in the past and incorporate them into the diet in moderation.
- Unless contraindicated, increase fluid intake.
- Increase activity level.
- Encourage the patient to develop good elimination habits, such as responding to physiologic cues for bowel movements and scheduling a regular time for elimination (e.g., after breakfast).

FAST FACTS in a NUTSHELL

Some older adults have incomplete emptying of the bowel and need to complete their bowel movement approximately 30 to 45 minutes after the initial bowel elimination. Patients and/or their caregivers should understand that a second use of the toilet may be necessary and schedule toileting time accordingly.

- Consult with the physician and pharmacist if medications are suspected as a contributing factor to constipation and explore alternatives.
- Teach techniques that facilitate bowel elimination, such as elevating the feet slightly and leaning forward to increase abdominal pressure.

- Utilize laxatives if other measures have not corrected the problem and monitor effects.
- Have the patient and/or caregivers monitor bowel elimination.

=== *FAST FACTS in a NUTSHELL*

A commode or commode chair is preferable to a bedpan for facilitating bowel elimination in a bedbound patient. A bedpan forces the extension of the legs, abdominal hyperextension, and defecation with minimal muscular help, thereby causing undue strain. In addition, if not properly positioned, gravity may impede the passage of stool.

Fecal Impaction

One of the complications of constipation is fecal impaction, the accumulation of feces in the rectum or colon that is difficult to pass. Factors that contribute to this problem include:

- Irregular bowel elimination
- Dehydration
- Decreased GI motility
- Impaired cognition
- Painful defecation related to anal fissures or hemorrhoids
- Sensory/motor disorders, such as cerebrovascular accident or neurological disease
- Lack of toileting assistance
- Side effects of medications (e.g., antacids, iron, calcium)

Fecal impaction can be apparent by:
- The absence of regular bowel movements
- Abdominal fullness and discomfort
- Distended rectum
- Oozing of fecal material from the rectum
- Poor appetite
- Lethargy
- Hard fecal mass, palpable with digital examination

FAST FACTS in a NUTSHELL

The oozing of fecal matter from the rectum that occurs with a fecal impaction can be easily mistaken for diarrhea. It is important to assess for other signs of fecal impaction when a patient has diarrhea to avoid misdiagnosis and inappropriate treatment.

Nurses should check with their organization's policies regarding the removal of fecal impaction. If this is an acceptable nursing procedure, the following actions are typically taken:

- Explain the procedure to the patient
- Position the patient on his or her left side with knees flexed and drape appropriately
- Ask the patient to take a deep breath to reduce the effects of Valsalva's maneuver
- Insert a lubricated gloved finger into the rectum and attempt to break up the mass before removing it
- Remove small masses of feces
- Talk with the patient throughout the procedure to promote relaxation
- Document results

Sometimes, manual removal is not effective and other measures are necessary to assist with the removal of the impaction, such as an oil-retention enema or the injection of 50 to 100 mL of hydrogen peroxide through a rectal tube.

Hemorrhoids

A hemorrhoid is a mass of dilated veins in swollen tissue near the anal sphincter that can be a chronic problem from earlier years or a new one in late life. Internal hemorrhoids develop above the anorectal line; external hemorrhoids occur below it. Chronic constipation, straining while defecating, and obesity are common causes. Clinical signs that will be present are:

- Perianal itching
- Bleeding during or after bowel movements

- Pain
- Swelling, bulges in rectal area
- Swollen, dilated perianal veins

Interventions will be aimed at relieving discomfort and reducing contributing factors, and could include:

- Warm sitz baths (due to older adults' more fragile tissue and susceptibility to burns, water temperature needs to be measured carefully)

FAST FACTS in a NUTSHELL

During a sitz bath, blood tends to be pulled to the lower extremities, which can lower blood pressure and cause dizziness. To prevent falls, close observation and support of the patient during the procedure are needed.

- Measures to prevent constipation
- Avoiding straining and sitting on toilet for long periods
- Use of witch hazel compresses after bowel movements for comfort

For severe cases of hemorrhoids, surgery may be recommended.

Diverticular Disease

Diverticulosis is a condition in which multiple pouches develop along the intestinal wall. This weakening of the muscular wall of the large bowel is a common condition among older adults. Obesity, low-residue diets, and age-related atrophy of the intestinal wall muscles contribute to this problem.

Typically, diverticulosis is asymptomatic; if symptoms develop they usually consist of slight bleeding, a change in bowel habits, and tenderness of the lower left quadrant when palpated. A barium enema will confirm the diagnosis and medical management, including increasing dietary fiber intake, weight reduction, and establishing a pattern of regular bowel elimination, is planned.

One of the risks with diverticulosis is that bowel contents can accumulate in the diverticula, decompose, and lead to inflammation and infection, known as diverticulitis. Signs of diverticulitis include:

- Pain in the lower left quadrant
- Nausea, vomiting
- Bowel irregularity (diarrhea, constipation, or both)
- Low-grade fever
- Mucus or blood in stool

FAST FACTS in a NUTSHELL

Acute attacks of diverticulitis can result in peritonitis; however, slowly progressing diverticulitis can be equally serious because it can lead to bowel obstruction due to scarring and abscess formation.

The goals during the acute phase include treating the infection, providing adequate nourishment (intravenously, if oral intake is contraindicated), and promoting comfort and rest. If medical management does not correct the problem, a colon resection or temporary colostomy may be required. The consequences of diverticulitis reinforce the importance of adequately managing diverticulosis to avoid this complication.

Colorectal Cancer

Colorectal cancer is among the leading malignancies in the United States, and the incidence increases with advancing age. In the early stages, the person may be asymptomatic, which emphasizes the importance of regular screening.

Symptoms can vary for each person but usually include:

- Change in bowel pattern
- Rectal bleeding, bloody stools
- Weight loss

- Anorexia, nausea
- Cramping abdominal pain
- Mucus discharge in feces

FAST FACTS in a NUTSHELL

Annual stool occult blood and digital rectal examinations are valuable aids in discovering colorectal cancers early. In addition, a flexible sigmoidoscopy every 5 years or a colonoscopy every 10 years is recommended.

When colorectal cancer is suspected, diagnostic testing is essential and can include a fecal occult blood test (FOBT), sigmoidoscopy, regular or standard colonoscopy, virtual colonoscopy, or double contrast barium enema (DCBE).

Typically, surgical resection with anastomosis or a colostomy is done.

FAST FACTS in a NUTSHELL

Although the basic care of a colostomy is the same for an older person as a younger one, arthritic fingers, reduced vision, and decreased energy are more likely to be present in the older adult and interfere with the ability to perform ostomy care. Altered body image and anxiety about being embarrassed if the bag should leak or having to be more dependent on others can interfere with the ability to manage the care of the ostomy. If dementia or other conditions are present, the self-care challenges are even greater. These factors must be assessed when helping the older adult adjust to and care for the ostomy.

6

Genitourinary System

Genitourinary conditions are common in late life, yet may be delayed in diagnosis due to the difficulty patients may have in discussing them. Further, some older adults may view incontinence, impotence, urinary frequency, and other signs of genitourinary disease as normal for persons their age. In addition to jeopardizing quality of life, these conditions can have serious health consequences; therefore, early identification and treatment are highly beneficial. Nurses can play an important role in helping older adults to have genitourinary conditions diagnosed and treated.

Objectives

In this chapter you will learn to:

1. Identify age-related changes to the genitourinary system
2. Describe components of the assessment of the genitourinary system
3. Differentiate normal from abnormal findings of the genitourinary system in late life

4. Describe the risk factors, symptoms, and care of the following conditions in older adults:
   - Urinary incontinence
   - Urinary tract infection (UTI)
   - Breast cancer
   - Vaginitis
   - Dyspareunia
   - Benign prostatic hyperplasia
   - Cancer of the prostate
   - Erectile dysfunction

AGE-RELATED CHANGES

A variety of changes impact the urinary tract with age, such as:

- Reduction in kidney size and renal tissue growth rate
- Reduction in renal blood flow
- Reduction in glomerular filtration rate by approximately one-half between the ages of 20 and 90 years (Lerma, 2009)
- Decreased tubular function, contributing to less efficient tubular exchange of substances, less conservation of water and sodium, and decreased reabsorption of glucose from the filtrate. As a result of these changes, 1+ proteinurias and 1+ glycosurias are not to be of major diagnostic significance and older adults can be hyperglycemic without experiencing

─────────────────── *FAST FACTS in a NUTSHELL*

Nocturia is a problem for older adults due to the changes in the bladder and the improvement in renal circulation that occurs when the person is in a recumbent position. They often need to void several hours after lying down and periodically during the night.

glycosuria. There also can be problems in the concentration of urine (the maximum specific gravity at 80 years of age is 1.024, whereas at younger ages it is 1.032)
- Weakening of bladder muscles, hypertrophy of bladder muscle, decreased ability to expand the bladder, and decreased bladder capacity, causing urinary frequency, urgency, and nocturia

- Incomplete emptying of the bladder resulting in urinary retention
- Delayed micturation reflex

=============== *FAST FACTS in a NUTSHELL*

Urinary incontinence is not a normal outcome of aging; however, many women experience stress incontinence due to a weakening of the pelvic diaphragm due to estrogen depletion or having experienced multiple pregnancies.

The reproductive system experiences multiple changes with age, as well. Changes to the female genitalia include:

- Atrophy of the vulva secondary to hormonal changes
- Loss of subcutaneous fat and hair and flattening of the labia
- Reduction in elasticity and secretions of vagina; thinner vaginal epithelium; more alkaline vaginal environment
- Shrinkage and atrophy of cervix; atrophy of endocervical epithelium
- Shrinkage of uterus, atrophy of endometrium; weakening of ligaments supporting the uterus (these factors can contribute to difficulty in palpating the uterus of older women)
- Atrophy and shortening of fallopian tubes
- Atrophy and shrinkage of ovaries

Despite these changes, older women are able to enjoy sex and experience orgasms.

After menopause the breasts sag and are less firm due to the replacement of mammary glands by fat tissue. Shrinkage and fibrotic changes to the nipples can result in their retraction to some extent.

Age-related changes to the male reproductive system include:

- Reduction in sperm count in some men due to increased fibrosis and narrowing of lumen of seminiferous tubules, and thinning of epithelium of seminal vesicles and seminiferous tubules
- Increase in FSH and LH levels; decreases in both serum and bioavailable testosterone levels

- Atrophy of testes
- Enlargement of prostate gland

Like the older woman, the older man does not lose the ability to enjoy sex and experience orgasm. He normally retains the ability to achieve erections or ejaculations, although orgasm and ejaculation tend to be less intense (Sampson, Untergasser, Plas, & Berger, 2007).

ASSESSMENT CONSIDERATIONS

Some older adults may have difficulty sharing that they experience incontinence, ejaculate prematurely, or cannot enjoy intercourse within a new relationship due to vaginal discomfort. They may have been socialized to believe these matters are private and not to be discussed with strangers, or believe that their sexual activity is abnormal for their age. Putting older adults at ease during the assessment and asking questions and accepting responses in a matter-of-fact manner can enable them to feel comfortable sharing symptoms and concerns. Examples of questions that could be asked during the interview to disclose problems of the urinary tract include:

- How often do you need to urinate during the day and during the night?
- Do you ever lose control of your urine? If so, please describe what that is like.
- Does your bladder ever feel full after you have urinated?
- Do you dribble urine after voiding?
- Has there been any recent change in the frequency or amount of urination, or characteristics of your urine?
- Do you have pain or burning when you urinate?
- Is your urine ever discolored? Does it ever have a strong odor, or have particles or blood in it? If so, please describe this.
- What prescription and over-the-counter medications are you using?
- What herbs and supplements are you using?

The presence of symptoms and a urine specimen yield considerable insights into conditions of the urinary system. When obtaining a urine specimen, note the color of the urine, particularly for:

- Dark coloration, which can occur with increased concentration, as occurs with dehydration
- Red or rust coloring, associated with the presence of blood
- Yellow-brown or green-brown color that can occur with jaundice or an obstructed bile duct
- Orange color, which reflects the presence of bile

The urine's specific gravity normally should range from 1.005 to 1.025, with a pH ranging from 4.6 to 8. Although not usually a normal finding, some glycosuria may be of no diagnostic significance.

Incorporating questions about sexual history and function in the assessment of the urinary system could be beneficial. Components of the sexual history of the older woman include:

- *Pregnancy history:* Attempt to outline year and outcome of each pregnancy. This can not only give insights into physical health problems, but also to emotional issues resulting from pregnancy and childbirth (e.g., depression over having had an abortion or inability to become pregnant).
- *Menstrual history:* Determine the onset and cessation of menstrual periods; review onset and experience with menopause.

FAST FACTS in a NUTSHELL

The American Cancer Society recommends annual mammograms and clinical breast exams for women age 40 and older until age 75, when mammograms can be reduced to every 2 years, providing there have been no abnormalities. Women with a high risk, such as those with a family history of breast cancer, should also be screened with MRI.

- *Gynecologic examination history and past problems*: Review the frequency of gynecologic exams and mammograms, and the dates of the last ones. Ask about significant events, such as abnormal findings, surgeries, or treatment for gynecologic conditions. Review the patient's knowledge of self-examination of the breasts.
- *Symptoms*: Ask about dyspareunia, vaginal bleeding or discharge, pelvic pressure or heaviness, breast lumps, nipple discharge, pain, and other symptoms.

A gynecologic examination should be arranged if the woman has not had one for more than 1 year. In addition to cancer, there are other conditions that can be discovered during the exam.

FAST FACTS in a NUTSHELL

The American College of Obstetricians and Gynecologists (2013) recommends an annual pelvic examination. Cervical cytology may be discontinued if the woman has had 3 or more consecutive normal test results, no abnormal test results in 10 years, no history of cervical cancer, no DES exposure in utero, is HIV-negative and immunocompetent, and does not have other risk factors for STDs.

The older male should be asked about concerns and symptoms related to the reproductive system and sexual function, including pain, impotency, discharge, bleeding, and unusual lumps. Most older men will have some enlargement of the prostate gland with related symptoms of urinary frequency, hesitancy, nocturia, dribbling, and less forceful ejaculations and urine stream. Most prostatic enlargement is benign, although the risk of prostate cancer does increase with age. Screening for prostate cancer includes:

- *Digital rectal examination*: This aids in determining the size of the gland and identifying lumps and other abnormalities. (Adhere to your organization's policy regarding the ability of nurses to perform digital rectal exams.)
- *Prostate-specific antigen (PSA) test*: An elevation in PSA occurs with prostate cancer; however, there are other factors that elevate the PSA, such as infection and certain medications. Routine PSA testing for men without a history of prostate cancer is not recommended.

Physical examination of the male genitalia begins with inspection of the penis for ulcers, chancres, nodules, and other abnormalities. If the patient is uncircumcised, pull back the foreskin and note any lesions and discharge that may be present. Inspect the scrotum for irritation, nodules, ulcers, and inflammation. Gently palpate the testes for lumps and enlargement. The patient should be referred for evaluation if abnormal findings are present.

=== *FAST FACTS in a NUTSHELL*

The American Cancer Society and Centers for Disease Control and Prevention, along with other federal agencies, recommend against PSA screening for men who do not have symptoms of prostate cancer.

CONDITIONS

Urinary Incontinence

The inability to control the release of urine increases in incidence with age. Despite urinary incontinence occurring more frequently in older adults as compared to other age groups, it is not a normal outcome of aging and requires evaluation to identify the cause and best treatment.

Incontinence can be *transient*, characterized by an abrupt onset and usually related to infections, medications, deliriums, mood disorders, fecal impactions, or the inability to reach or use a commode or urinal. Incontinence related to these causes can be reversed by addressing the underlying cause.

Established incontinence, which is chronic in nature, can appear abruptly or slowly and includes the following types:

- *Stress*: weakness of the supporting pelvic muscles causes urine to be released through the bladder outlet during coughing, laughing, sneezing, or exercising.
- *Urgency*: spasm or irritation of bladder walls, causing a sudden need to void and involuntary passage of urine due to UTIs, enlarged prostate, diverticulitis, or bladder or pelvic tumors.

- *Neurogenic (reflex):* lack of sensation to the signal to void that leads to involuntary loss of urine when a specific volume of urine fills the bladder; caused by disturbances along the neural pathway (e.g., multiple sclerosis, cerebral cortex lesions).
- *Overflow:* excess accumulation of urine in the bladder that results in involuntary release due to overflow; associated with bladder neck obstructions, neurogenic conditions of the bladder, or medications (e.g., adrenergics, anticholinergics, calcium channel blockers).
- *Functional:* existence of factors that interfere with the ability to reach or use a toilet, bedpan, or urinal; can occur due to cognitive impairment, sedation, immobility, lack of assistance in toileting, or inaccessible bathroom.

In some circumstances, incontinence can arise from a combination of factors; this is referred to as mixed incontinence.

FAST FACTS in a NUTSHELL

There are circumstances in which incontinence, even long-term incontinence, has not been fully evaluated and a reversible cause has not been identified and treated. Nurses need to ask about this problem during the assessment and advocate for the proper diagnostic testing and treatment.

Patients should be asked about the presence of urinary incontinence during the assessment. If a positive response is offered, questions should be asked concerning:

- Date of onset and anything that occurred at that time that could have contributed (e.g., UTI, hospitalization, new prescription)
- Patterns (e.g., sudden expulsion of large amounts of urine, constant dribbling)
- Frequency and occurrence (e.g., only at night, when sneezing)
- Precipitating factors (e.g., using diuretics, laughing, delayed voiding)
- Related factors (e.g., weight gain, constipation, new medications)
- Typical diet (caffeine, citrus fruits, spicy foods, and artificial sweeteners can be bladder irritants)
- Intake and output

- Reactions (e.g., embarrassment, reduced socialization, acceptance)
- Other symptoms (e.g. abdominal pain, fever)

Review the medical history for conditions that could contribute to incontinence, such as dementia, cerebrovascular accident, UTI, and diabetes mellitus. Review prescription and nonprescription medications being used.

===== *FAST FACTS in a NUTSHELL*

Medications that affect continence include diuretics, antianxiety agents, antipsychotics, antidepressants, sedatives, narcotics, antiparkinsonism agents, antispasmodics, antihistamines, calcium channel blockers, alpha-blockers, and alpha-stimulants.

Cognition and mood should be assessed to determine their influence on continence.

Physical assessment is invaluable to the diagnostic process and includes assessment of:

- *Bladder fullness and pain*: percuss and palpate the bladder noting sensitivity, distention, and abnormalities
- *Lower extremity neuromuscular function*: touch various areas along both legs with a pin point to determine the patient's ability to feel; touch various areas along both legs with the pin point and smooth side of a safety pin to determine the patient's ability to differentiate sensations; ask the patient to lift his or her leg and keep it lifted as you try to gently push it down

Positive findings may warrant diagnostic tests such as urinalysis, cystoscopy, cystometrogram, and cystometry.

The factor responsible for the incontinence will determine the treatment, and in some circumstances, as with an infection, the problem could be corrected. When incontinence is not transient, interventions that could be used include:

- Monitoring intake and output
- Providing easily accessible toilet facilities; arrange for urinal or bedside commode if necessary. Assist as needed.

- Determining the effectiveness of a toileting program and implementing the most appropriate one; this could include:
  - *Timed voiding:* Through the use of a voiding record the anticipated times for voiding are identified and toileting times scheduled for a short time prior to the anticipated voiding time. This works best for patients who do not have physical or cognitive disabilities.

FAST FACTS in a NUTSHELL

As measuring urinary output of the person who is incontinent can be challenging, one means of estimating output is by equating one inch of an area of wet clothing or linens to 10 mL of urine.

- *Prompted voiding:* The person is asked, prior to anticipated time for voiding, to void and is assisted in doing so. Praise is offered if the person has remained dry between scheduled voiding.
- *Pelvic floor strengthening (Kegel) exercises:* The woman is aided in identifying the pelvic floor muscles by asking her to stop the flow of urine while voiding and noticing the tightening of the muscles in the vaginal area and lifting of the pelvic floor, or to insert a finger into the vagina, tighten the muscles around the finger, and notice the effect on muscles and the pelvic floor. Instruct her to tighten these muscles for 10 seconds and then relax for 10 seconds before repeating for 10 sets of exercises. These should be repeated daily, several times throughout the day. It can take several weeks to several months for results to be noted.
- Using Crede's maneuver: For patients with incomplete bladder emptying or overflow, manual compressing over the suprapubic area during voiding will aid in bladder emptying.
- Teaching self-catheterization, if indicated, and helping the patient obtain necessary equipment. Arrange for a home health nursing referral as needed.
- Referring the patient for biofeedback training if deemed a good candidate.
- Supporting pharmacological therapies.

- Assisting with the use of effective containment measures, such as adult briefs, urinary sheaths, and condom catheters. Avoid indwelling catheter use due to the high risk for infection.
- Teaching community-based persons about methods and resources to protect the mattress, control odors, and avoid falls.
- Monitoring skin status.
- Taking precautions to avoid falls (e.g., cleaning urine spills promptly, keeping a clear path to the bathroom, providing adequate lighting for nighttime trips to the bathroom).

FAST FACTS in a NUTSHELL

Nurses can significantly affect the quality of life of older adults who are incontinent by ensuring the condition is properly evaluated and treated, rather than assumed to be a normal outcome of aging, and that the person is treated with dignity.

Urinary Tract Infection (UTI)

UTIs increase in incidence with age and are the most common infection of older adults. Persons at risk for UTI are those who have fluid imbalances, urethral strictures, diabetes, neurogenic bladders, and poor toileting hygenic practices, as well as those who are immobile, have been frequently catheterized, or have an indwelling catheter.

FAST FACTS in a NUTSHELL

Most UTIs are caused by Escherichia coli in women and Proteus species in men.

Clinical signs of UTI include:

- Urinary frequency, urgency
- Burning sensation when voiding
- Incontinence
- Delirium
- As it advances: hematuria, retention
  Bacteriuria greater than 105 CFU/mL confirms the diagnosis.

FAST FACTS in a NUTSHELL

Some of the classic signs of UTI can be missed in the older adult.

[Clinical Snapshot]

Seventy-eight-year-old assisted living resident, Ms. J, complained of having to void frequently. Her caregivers took her temperature and found it to be 98.8°F, so they assured her there was no problem but that frequent voiding was normal for someone her age. Unfortunately, they had not reviewed her medical record to see that her usual body temperature was 97.6°F. It wasn't until several days later when her temperature increased to 100°F and her urine became cloudy and odorous that a specimen was obtained and her UTI diagnosed.

In males, prostatitis is the most common UTI. Symptoms include frequency, nocturia, dysuria, and varying degrees of bladder obstruction secondary to an edematous, enlarged prostate, as well as lower back and perineal pain. Acute prostatitis usually responds well to antibiotic therapy; chronic prostatitis responds less to antibiotics and is more difficult to treat.

Antibiotic therapy is ordered to control the infection. The nurse should support this therapy and:

- Force fluids, unless contraindicated
- Monitor intake and output
- Instruct the patient in proper hygienic practices if this was found to be a problem
- Observe for worsening of symptoms that could indicate urosepsis (septicemia secondary to UTI)

As indwelling urinary catheters carry a significant risk for causing UTI, nurses should discourage their use.

Breast Cancer

Breast cancer is the second leading cause of cancer deaths for women, with about half of the new cases diagnosed in older women.

Women should be routinely asked about the dates of their last mammogram and their breast self-examination practices. Instruction on self-examination should be provided if the woman does not understand the correct procedure. (The American Cancer Society offers breast examination guides that can be useful. Information can be obtained at local chapters or www.cancer.org.)

Risk factors for breast cancer include beginning to menstruate before age 12, late menopause, having the first full-term pregnancy after age 30, high fat intake, obesity, having dense breasts, and high alcohol consumption. Inherited alterations in the BRCA1 and BRCA2 (short for *breast cancer 1 and breast cancer 2*) genes are involved in many cases of hereditary breast cancer. The risk that BRCA1 or BRCA2 is associated with these cancers is highest in women with a family history of multiple cases of breast cancer, with at least one family member having two primary cancers at different sites, or who are of Eastern European (Ashkenazi) Jewish background (American Cancer Society, 2012).

FAST FACTS in a NUTSHELL

According to the Centers for Disease Control and Prevention (2013), Black women have the highest death rates from breast cancer of all racial and ethnic groups, and are 40% more likely to die from this disease as compared to White women. More aggressive cancers experienced by Black women and disparities in health care are among the factors contributing to this difference.

The classic signs of breast cancer are:

- Breast mass or lump
- Asymmetry of breasts
- Dimpling of skin (orange-peel appearance)
- Nipple changes, discharge, or bleeding

If the disease has progressed, pain, weight loss, and generalized weakness can be present. As breast cancer typically is asymptomatic in its early stage, regular mammography is extremely beneficial to early detection.

In addition to mammograms, diagnostic tests include magnetic resonance imaging, breast ultrasound, and surgical biopsy. If nipple discharge is present, a ductogram may be performed, in which a thin plastic tube is placed in the opening of the duct in the nipple, a contrast medium is injected, and an x-ray is done, which outlines the duct and reveals any mass that is present. After it is diagnosed, the cancer is staged based on whether it has invaded the body or is noninvasive, tumor size, number of lymph nodes involved, and metastasis.

A mastectomy can require longer a longer period of recovery for the older woman. It is important that the arm on the operative side be exercised through a full range of motion to prevent lymphedema of the arm. Guidance should be offered as to obtaining a prosthesis. Of upmost importance is emotional support. The woman should be encouraged to express her feelings and any misconceptions should be clarified. Referring her to a local support group is beneficial.

Vaginitis

Atrophy and thinning of vaginal tissues, increased alkalinity of the secretions, and reduced lubrication contribute to a risk for vaginitis in older women. Vaginal symptoms can include:

- Soreness
- Pruritus
- Burning
- Redness
- Discharge (often foul smelling)

Topical estrogens usually are effective in treating this infection. It is useful to advise women to wear cotton underwear and avoid douching and the use of feminine deodorants or perfumes. If they use a lubricant to ease penile penetration during intercourse, advise them to use a water-soluble one (e.g., K-Y gel).

FAST FACTS in a NUTSHELL

Some older women may feel embarrassed that their vaginitis is related to their sexual activity. Introducing the topic and discussing sexual activity and tips for comfortable, safe sex in a matter-of-fact manner can imply that it is neither unusual nor inappropriate for them to engage in sexual activity.

Dyspareunia

Painful intercourse, dyspareunia, can be experienced by older women as a result of changes to their reproductive system. The problem is more common in women who have not had children. Sufficient foreplay and a water-soluble vaginal lubricant can aid in lubricating the vagina and easing penile penetration. If these measures do not relieve the discomfort, a gynecologic examination may be beneficial to ensure vaginitis, vulvitis, or other conditions are not present.

Benign Prostatic Hyperplasia

A noncancerous enlargement of the prostate gland is present in most older men and can be palpated upon digital rectal examination. As the gland enlarges pressure is placed on the urethra, resulting in symptoms such as:

- Hesitancy
- Decreased force of urinary stream
- Urinary frequency, nocturia
- Dribbling of urine, poor control of urine release
- Bleeding
- UTI

Some men may be hesitant to contribute that these symptoms are present, so asking specifically about them can prove useful in identifying the problem.

Prostatic massage and urinary antiseptics are among the major treatments for benign prostatic hyperplasia. As diuretics, anticholinergics, and antiarrhythmic agents can contribute to the problem, alternatives to them should be considered, if possible. In some cases, prostatectomy may be done. This surgery does not necessarily result in impotence, so men should not hesitate to have the surgery for that reason.

Cancer of the Prostate

Prostate cancer increases in incidence with age. Although evidence of cancer in the prostate gland is present in more than half of the men over age 70, less than 3% will die from the disease (National

Cancer Institute, 2013). A majority of these cancers can be discovered through digital rectal examination, along with a positive PSA test. Symptoms can be similar to those associated with benign prostatic hyperplasia. If the disease metastasizes, anemia, weakness, weight loss, and back pain may be present. The diagnosis is confirmed through biopsy.

The National Cancer Institute (2013), based on the results of clinical trials, suggests that men with early-stage prostate cancer can live as long without surgery as men who have immediate surgery. Men with high-grade, aggressive prostate cancers do benefit from surgery and radiation.

Erectile Dysfunction

Although not a normal outcome of aging, the inability to achieve and/or sustain an erection for intercourse is a common problem in men over age 70. Factors that increase the risk of this problem include alcoholism, diabetes, dyslipidemia, hypertension, hypogonadism, multiple sclerosis, renal failure, spinal cord injury, and thyroid conditions. Psychological factors also can contribute to erectile dysfunction, as can some medications (e.g., anticholinergics, antidepressants, antihypertensives, digoxin, sedatives, and tranquilizers). Treatment for erectile dysfunction can include:

- Oral erectile agents: sildenafil citrate (Viagra), vardenafil HCl (Levitra), tadalafil (Cialis)
- Drugs injected in the penis
- Penile implants
- Vacuum pump devices

FAST FACTS in a NUTSHELL

A comprehensive patient evaluation needs to be done before erectile agents are used, as these drugs carry serious risks and are contraindicated for some individuals. Men should be cautioned not to obtain or use these medications without an evaluation by their health care provider.

7

Musculoskeletal System

Be it muscles that become sore from the same degree of activity that didn't cause soreness in younger years, joints that are stiff upon awakening, or changes in body strength and shape, the impact of age on the musculoskeletal system is not that difficult to notice. The challenge is that the effects of aging on the musculoskeletal system can cause individuals to reduce activity; in turn, reduced activity can make the effects of aging more pronounced and further limit activity. Measures to maximize movement and promote musculoskeletal function are important to every older adult.

Objectives

In this chapter you will learn to:

1. Identify age-related changes to the musculoskeletal system
2. Describe components of the assessment of the musculoskeletal system

3. Recognize the clinical signs and describe the care of older patients with:
   • Osteoporosis
   • Osteoarthritis
   • Rheumatoid arthritis
   • Gout
   • Fractures
   • Podiatric conditions

AGE-RELATED CHANGES

A variety of changes occur within the musculoskeletal system, many of which are noticeable in terms of appearance and function. These include:

• Atrophy and reduction in muscle fiber
• Decrease in muscle mass, strength, and movement
• Loss of motor neurons
• Reduction in bone mineral and mass
• Decrease in bone density of about 0.5% per year after the third decade
• Reduced calcium absorption
• Slower production of new bone secondary to decreased osteoblastic production of bone matrix
• Increased bone resorption
• Deterioration of intervertebral discs
• Deterioration of cartilage surface of joints
• Decline in strength of tendons and ligaments
• Degeneration of collagen and elastin cells
• Shrinkage and hardening of tendons, decrease in tendon jerks
• Reduced reflexes in arms and abdomen

Older individuals often detect these changes through a reduction in height, poor muscle tone, slight kyphosis, and enlarged joints. Joint pain, weaker muscles, and muscle cramping are also reminders of these changes.

=== *FAST FACTS in a NUTSHELL*

Engaging in regular exercise can aid in slowing or preventing many of the changes to musculoskeletal system, in addition to offering benefits to other body systems.

ASSESSMENT CONSIDERATIONS

Assessment of the musculoskeletal system begins upon first observation of the patient. Observe the patient's posture and how the patient walks, moves, sits, and talks. Note abnormalities of structure, such as asymmetry or misalignment of body parts, and movement, such as abnormal gait, tremor, redness or swelling of a joint, reduced or lack of function of a limb, and weakness. If the patient uses a cane, walker, or wheelchair, question the reason and length of use and note if the aid is used correctly.

Much about musculoskeletal function and symptoms is gained through a structured interview. Specific questions that could be asked include:

- Do you feel any pain in your bones, muscles, or joints? If so, what causes it and what makes it better?
- Do you ever have difficulty moving your legs or arms? Turning your head? Bending? If so, when does this happen, what seems to cause it, and what makes it better?
- After walking, do your feet hurt? Your legs? Your hips?
- Do you ever have back pain or stiffness? If so, what causes this, how long does it last, and what makes it better?
- Do you have muscles cramps? If so, what causes them, how long do they last, and what makes them better?
- How far are you able to walk?
- Do bone, muscle, or joint pain symptoms interfere with your ability to care for yourself or participate in activities?
- On a scale of 1 to 10, with 1 being not active at all and 10 being extremely active, how would you rate your activity level?

• Do you use medications to prevent or treat bone, muscle, or joint pain? If so, what do you use, how often, what dose, and with what results?
• Do you use any herbs, heat, cold, or other measures to manage symptoms of your bones, muscles, or joints?

Evaluating range of motion is a major component of the physical assessment. Table 7.1 describes the expected range of motion. Deviations from the normal should be described as specifically as possible.

TABLE 7.1 Assessing Range of Motion

Joint	Normal Range of Motion
Neck	Ability for 30° lateral turn, extension, and flexion of head
Shoulder	Ability to move straight arm from relaxed position at side, forward, and overhead to 160° angle Ability to extend straight arms from sides to behind body to 30° angle with body
Elbow	Ability of the hand to swing back to touch shoulder from full-arm extension
Wrist	From position of being perpendicular with floor, the wrist should rotate 90° to each side From parallel to ground, wrist should flex downward 80° and upward 70° From parallel with ground, the wrist should move 10° toward radial or thumb side and 60° toward ulnar side
Finger	Distal phalange should bend 45°, proximal joint should bend 90°
Thumb	Distal portion should bend 90°, proximal portion should bend 70°
Hip	From supine position, leg should rise toward chin 90° with leg straight and 125° with knee bent From prone position, leg should extend backward 5° From straight alignment with body, leg should abduct 45° and adduct 45°

(continued)

TABLE 7.1 **Assessing Range of Motion** (continued)	
Joint	**Normal Range of Motion**
Knee	From prone position, knee should be able to flex 100°
Ankle	Should be able to flex toes toward head (dorsiflexion) 10° and extend toward floor or foot of bed (plantar flexion) 40° Should be able to turn foot inward (inversion) 35° and turn outward (eversion) 25°
Toe	Should be able to flex and extend toes approximately 30°

=== *FAST FACTS in a NUTSHELL*

Sarcopenia is the decline in the size and number of skeletal muscle fibers and the loss of muscle mass and strength that occurs with age. The result is increased muscle weakness, ease of muscle fatigue, reduced tolerance for exercise, less stable gait, increased risk of falls, and a greater risk of disability. In addition to the aging process, inactivity, protein deficiency, and weight loss contribute to the development of sarcopenia (Jones et al., 2009). Good protein intake, physical activity, and strength training can prevent and reverse sarcopenia.

Although it will vary, even among individuals of the same age, some weakening of muscles can be an anticipated finding with older adults. Palpate all muscles, noting tenderness, masses, and contractures. Inspect the body for muscle atrophy. A gross testing of muscle strength can be done by asking the patient to flex the limb and applying force to extend the muscle. The patient should be able to maintain flexion against moderate force. Typically, greater strength is present in the arm of the dominant hand; the strength in the lower extremities should be equal. If unusual muscle weakness is noted without justification from the medical history, refer the patient for further evaluation.

CONDITIONS

Osteoporosis

Osteoporosis, the most prevalent metabolic disease of the bone, causes a reduction in the mineral and protein matrix of bones that results in diffuse reduction of bone density. The reduced bone density allows bones to fracture under minimal stress.

The high prevalence of osteoporosis in the older population is not surprising when the causative and contributing factors are considered; these include:

- Deficiency of calcium and vitamin D
- Inactivity or immobility, which causes high rates of bone resorption
- Estrogen and androgen deficiencies
- Diseases, such as diabetes mellitus, Cushing syndrome, chronic diverticulitis, and hyperthyroidism
- Medications such as aluminum- and magnesium-based antacids, corticosteroids, heparin, furosemide
- Cigarette smoking
- High alcohol consumption
- Small bone structure
- Family history of osteoporosis

=========================== *FAST FACTS in a NUTSHELL*

Osteoporosis can be present although not formally diagnosed. Sometimes, the condition is not identified and treated until a fracture occurs. It is advantageous to suggest screening for osteoporosis in older adults who are at risk in an effort to identify the condition and take action to prevent fractures.

Asian and White women with a northwestern European or British Isles background, as well as women over 65 years and men over 80 years, are at high risk for developing this disease.

Many patients with osteoporosis are asymptomatic. If symptoms are present they can include a reduction in height, kyphosis, spinal pain, and ease of bone fracture. The most widely used method for diagnosing osteoporosis is dual-energy x-ray absorptiometry (DEXA). Other measures to measure bone mass include single-photon absorptiometry (SPA), dual-photon absorptiometry (DPA), and quantitative computed tomography (CT).

The underlying factor responsible for the development of the disease will determine the treatment and could include calcium supplements, vitamin D supplements, progesterone, estrogen, anabolic agents, fluoride, or phosphate. A synthetic form of calcitonin can be prescribed to increase bone mass, as can drugs of the bisphosphonate group, which prevent or slow bone resorption. Nurses should instruct patients to take caution to prevent fractures; this includes avoiding heavy lifting, jumping, and engaging in activities in which the bones may be bumped. Physical exercise to improve gait and balance and range of motion exercises are beneficial. Caregivers should be advised to handle the patient gently, taking care not to have limbs hit siderails or to allow the patient to be "dropped" into place when lifting into a chair or wheelchair. Keeping the bed in the lowest position and placing mats around the bed will reduce the impact of a fall from bed and could aid in preventing a fracture.

Osteoarthritis

The progressive degenerative inflammatory disease of the joints and attached muscles, tendons, and ligaments—osteoarthritis—is the leading cause of physical disability in the older population. Overuse of the joint, obesity, genetic factors, trauma to the joint, and low levels of vitamins D and C contribute to this problem. These factors worsen the age-related joint changes that result from a lack of homeostasis (due to the imbalance between destructive [matrix metalloprotease enzymes] and synthetic [tissue inhibitors of matrix metalloprotease] elements) that is necessary to maintain the cartilage. Common sites that are affected are the fingers, knees, hips, and vertebrae.

Symptoms are confined to the affected joint and include pain (particularly during movement and weight bearing), joint stiffness, crepitation on joint movement, and the development of bony nodules (Heberden nodes) over the joint. Symptoms may worsen during periods of overuse of the joint or weather changes.

A variety of approaches are used in the care of patients with osteoarthritis:

- Joint pain is typically managed with the use of analgesics, with acetaminophen as the first drug of choice because of its safety over nonsteroidal anti-inflammatory drugs (NSAIDs).
- Rest and gentle massage of the joint can be comforting. For some patients heat brings relief, while the application of cold is effective for others.
- A diet rich in essential fatty acids is beneficial due to their anti-inflammatory effects.
- Weight reduction often aids in relieving joint stress and reducing discomfort.

FAST FACTS in a NUTSHELL

Alternative and complementary therapies such as tai chi, acupuncture, and glucosamine and chondroitin supplements are beneficial for some people with osteoarthritis.

[Clinical Snapshot]

At the end of a class on the topic of arthritis that a nurse is presenting to a group at a senior citizen center, one of the participants stands and says to the group, "Those medicines and exercises aren't anywhere near as good as the supplement I buy from my neighbor. And, because it's natural, it has got to be safer." While acknowledging that there are some natural products that can be helpful, the nurse cautions the group that not all claims of products promoted for arthritis are based on sound research, and that natural doesn't necessarily mean safe. The nurse recommends that prior to using any alternative or complementary therapy for any purpose, it is wise to discuss the use of these therapies with one's health care provider to ensure there are no contraindications.

- Good body mechanics and proper body alignment can aid in promoting comfort and reducing the risk of further disability.
- To promote independent function, the patient can be referred to physical and occupational therapists for assistive devices.
- In some circumstances, when discomfort and joint function limitations are significant, arthroplasty, or joint replacement, can be done. Hip and knee joint replacements are the most common. Patients who have the physical and mental ability to participate in rehabilitation are the best candidates for this procedure. Certain conditions (e.g., diabetes mellitus, peripheral vascular disease) increase the risk for infection with this surgery, therefore, special precautions are warranted. As deep venous thrombosis (DVT) and pulmonary embolism are particular risks for older adults undergoing joint replacement, an anticoagulant may be used prophylactically. Patients and their caregivers should be instructed in the precautions related to anticoagulant therapy. Physical therapy usually will provide specific instructions related to weight-bearing activity and exercise; nurses should reinforce these instructions and ensure they are understood and adhered to by patients and their caregivers.

Rheumatoid Arthritis

Although it does not affect as many older adults as osteoarthritis and decreases in incidence with age, rheumatoid arthritis is a major cause of disability in late life and is a serious problem due to its deforming and debilitating effects. Most individuals with this form of arthritis developed it during early adulthood, particularly during the third and fourth decades of life when the incidence peaks. This disease affects women more than men and persons with a family history are more susceptible.

Rheumatoid arthritis causes the affected joints to become painful, red, swollen, and stiff. This is a result of the synovium becoming hypertrophied and edematous; synovial tissue also protrudes into the joint cavity. Subcutaneous nodules develop over bony prominences and there is atrophy of the surrounding muscles. As the disease progresses, flexion contractures develop, compounding the disability. Unlike osteoarthritis, rheumatoid arthritis creates systemic symptoms, including fatigue, malaise, weakness, anorexia, weight loss, wasting, fever, and anemia.

Examination of synovial fluid and x-rays help in the diagnosis. Laboratory evaluation of blood shows an elevated sedimentation rate and erythrocyte count during attacks.

================================ *FAST FACTS in a NUTSHELL*

Persons with rheumatoid arthritis may have sensitivity to the "nightshade" foods, such as potatoes, peppers, eggplant, and tomatoes. Eliminating these foods from the diet could aid in reducing symptoms.

The treatment plan can consist of:

- Rest and support to the affected limb.
- The use of splints to prevent deformities.
- Medications, such as anti-inflammatory agents (particularly prostaglandins), corticosteroids, antimalarial agents, gold salts, and immunosuppressive drugs. As these medications carry the potential for serious adverse effects for older adults, close monitoring of their effects is essential.
- Referral to physical and occupational therapists for various assistive devices that can ease and promote self-care independence.
- Range of motion exercises to promote musculoskeletal function.
- The use of heat to promote comfort.
- Elimination of "nightshade" foods as sensitivity is known to exist.

Gout

Gout is a metabolic disorder in which overproduction or underexcretion of uric acid causes excess uric acid to accumulate in the blood and ultimately deposit uric acid crystals in and around the joints. The crystals cause severe pain and tenderness of the joint, and swelling, redness, and warmth of the surrounding tissue. The joint at the base of the great toe is the most common site for a gout attack. During an attack the pain can be so severe that even a sheet rubbing against the affected joint can cause severe pain. Gout attacks can last from weeks to months; fortunately, there can be long periods of remission in between attacks.

In addition to symptoms, the diagnosis of gout can be made through examination of synovial fluid, which will show urate crystals and high levels of uric acid in the blood.

During acute attacks, colchicine or phenylbutazone prove helpful. Colchicine, allopurinol, probenecid, or indomethacin may be used for long-term management of gout. A good fluid intake should be encouraged to assist in the prevention of renal stones. Vitamin E, folic acid, and eicosapentaenoic acid (EPA) are dietary supplements that are beneficial to some patients with the condition. It is beneficial to avoid pressure on the joint (e.g., using a cane if the toe is affected) and to elevate the joint. Ice packs can relieve pain and inflammation.

Persons with gout should avoid substances that raise uric acid levels in the blood, such as:

- Thiazide diuretics
- Alcohol
- Foods high in purine, including bacon, turkey, veal, liver, kidney, brain, anchovies, sardines, herring, smelt, mackerel, salmon, and legumes

Fractures

In addition to a fragility of the bones that increases their ability to fracture, older adults often have conditions and impairments that increase their risk of falling, such as unsteady gait, weakness, medication side effects, urinary frequency, postural hypotension, vision impairments, and altered mood or cognition. Like younger adults, older adults can experience fractures from a forceful impact; however, unlike younger persons, older individuals can experience fractures with little to no impact.

The most common site of fractures in older adults is the neck of the femur, and most of these fractures are the result of falls. Colles' fracture (distal radius) is the most common upper extremity fall. Compression fractures of the vertebrae are another common site and can occur due to falls, heavy lifting, or being "dropped" into a chair during the last few inches of a transfer.

In addition to having their bones fracture more easily, older adults take longer to heal from fractures and experience more complications as they do. This emphasizes the importance of promoting safety to prevent falls and other incidents that could lead to fractures. Tips to offer older adults include:

- Wear safe, properly fitting shoes
- Change positions slowly
- Hold on to railings when on stairs
- Place both feet near the edge of a curb or high step before stepping, rather than stretching the legs over a large area
- Use sunglasses when outdoors in the sun
- Keep a nightlight on in the bathroom
- Avoid climbing ladders or standing on chairs to reach high areas
- Examine surfaces before walking on them for slippery or uneven areas

FAST FACTS in a NUTSHELL

According to the Centers for Disease Control and Prevention (2013), one in every three persons over age 65 experiences a fall annually. In addition to being a common cause of injuries and trauma-related hospital admissions for older adults, falls are the leading cause of injury death for this population.

A fracture should be suspected whenever an older adults falls or suffers a traumatic impact. Symptoms consistent with a fracture include:

- Pain
- Change in length or shape of limb
- Swelling
- Discoloration of affected area
- Protrusion of bone through the skin

Patients should be immobilized until evaluated for fracture. It is best to be cautious and refer the patient for an x-ray and further evaluation if there is any suspicion of an injury. The fact that symptoms are absent does not necessarily mean that there is no fracture.

Sometimes as the patient moves the fracture becomes apparent; therefore, close observation of the patient for several hours following a fall or other trauma is beneficial.

Podiatric Conditions

A majority of older adults have some type of foot problem, the most common being:

- *Calluses (plantar keratoses):* layers of thickened skin caused by chronic friction and irritation. They typically develop on an area that normally has thick skin, such as the heels and soles of the feet. The regular use of lotions and oils can keep the skin soft and aid in avoiding callus formation.
- *Corns:* a red, dry, thickened piece of skin usually found over a bony prominence of the toe that develops due to pressure. The corn is cone-shaped, with the tip of the cone pointing inward and leading to pain when pressure is placed on it. U-shaped pads are effective in relieving pressure while not reducing circulation to the area, as can occur with round or oval pads.
- *Bunions (Hallux valgus):* a structural deformity in which there is medial deviation of the first metatarsal and abduction of the great toe in relation to that metatarsal. A bursa (bunion) may form at the medial side of the metatarsal. Most bunions result from chronic wearing of tight fitting shoes and stockings. Having shoes stretched or obtaining custom-made shoes may help to accommodate the increased width of the foot; in some cases, surgery may be necessary.
- *Plantar fasciitis:* an inflammation of the thick ligamentous band that is located from the heel (where it is attached) to the ball of the foot caused by poor alignment of the foot. Heel pain occurs and is usually worse after a period of rest and when pressure is placed on the heel. Stretching exercises consisting of pulling up on the ball of the foot, applying ice for short periods, and wearing custom-made orthotics can provide relief, although it can take months for results to be noted.
- *Hammer toe (digiti flexus):* named this due to its resemblance to the shape of hammers inside a piano, this structural deformity is a hyperextension at the metatarsophalangeal joint with flexion and often corn formation at the proximal

interphalangeal joint. Although some symptomatic relief can be obtained by the use of orthotics, surgery is the means to correct this problem.

- *Athlete's foot (tinea pedis):* a fungal infection of the foot causing burning, itching, redness, and peeling of the skin. Vesicle eruptions may be noted. The dryness and cracking of the skin can cause breaks in the skin's integrity, thereby permitting bacteria to enter and further aggravate the problem.
- *Toenail problems:* Thickening of the toenails, onychauxis, is a common occurrence among older adults and can make toenail cutting challenging. Thick, enlarged, flaky, and brittle nails can indicate a fungal infection, known as onychomycosis; as the fungus grows under the nail it raises the nail and pushes the sides of the nail into the skin, causing pain. Onycholysis is a loosening of the nail at its distal portion, which can cause discomfort and self-image problems. Ingrown nails, onychocryptosis, can pierce the skin and cause infection.

FAST FACTS in a NUTSHELL

It is not unusual for people to try to shave or cut off their corns and calluses, which can cause infection and injury to the foot. Patients need to be advised about the risks associated with these practices and instructed on good foot care measures.

When foot conditions are identified, ask the patient about symptoms and care of them. It is useful to instruct the patient in good foot care practices, such as keeping feet clean and dry, applying moisturizing lotions, wearing safe properly fitting shoes, cutting toenails even with the top of the toe, avoiding tight-fitting shoes and stockings, not going barefoot, and exercising feet. Refer to a podiatrist as needed.

Safety, comfort, and function are major factors that have a significant impact on quality of life. These are also factors that are impacted by musculoskeletal conditions. By helping older adults to promote musculoskeletal health and identify signs of and properly treat musculoskeletal conditions, nurses can enable older adults to be maximally independent.

8

Neurological System

The neurological system functions to help us receive, process, and respond to information. Healthy function of this system impacts our communication with the environment and its many components, both in terms of our perception of the world around us and the appropriateness of our responses based on those responses. Our ability to protect ourselves from harm, engage in intellectually stimulating activities, accurately perceive reality, enjoy the pleasures of the environment, and react in a normal manner rely on the status of the neurological system. Age-related changes and diseases that affect this system, therefore, can have a profound impact on health, function, and quality of life.

Objectives

In this chapter you will learn to:

1. Identify age-related changes to the neurological system
2. Describe components of the assessment of the neurological system
3. Recognize the clinical signs and describe the care of older patients with:

- Cataracts
- Glaucoma
- Macular degeneration
- Detached retina
- Hearing deficits
- Transient ischemic attacks
- Cerebrovascular accident (CVA)
- Parkinson's disease

AGE-RELATED CHANGES

The impact of aging on the neurological system is difficult to determine because the status of this system is dependent on many other factors, such as lifestyle behaviors, diet, genetic composition, and the status of other systems. There are some changes that generally occur, such as:

- Reduction in neurons. Each neuron has fewer dendrites and experiences some demyelinization, which slow nerve conduction
- Slower response and reaction times
- Decreased cerebral blood flow, glucose utilization, and oxygen metabolism in brain
- Presence of beta-amyloid and neurofibrillary tangles (although present with Alzheimer's disease, they are present in persons with normal cognitive function)
- Decrease in brain weight and size
- Less effective temperature regulation by hypothalamus
- Less prominent stages III and IV of sleep
- Duller tactile sensation due to decrease in number and sensitivity of sensory receptors and dermatomes
- Less acute sense of taste and smell due to declining function of cranial nerves mediating these senses
- Development of presbyopia, the inability to focus or accommodate properly due to reduced elasticity of the lens resulting in farsightedness and reduced ability to adapt to light
- Narrowing of the visual field
- Less pupil response to light due to reduction in pupil size and hardening of pupil sphincter; increased difficulty with vision in dim areas or at night

- Opacity of lens leading to development of cataracts, which causes blurring of vision, increasing sensitivity to glare, and difficulty with night vision
- Yellowing of lens and retinal changes that create difficulty in perceiving low-tone colors (e.g., blues, greens, and violets)
- Altered depth perception
- Increased risk for glaucoma due to less efficient reabsorption of intraocular fluid
- Reduced lacrimal secretions
- Development of arcus senilis (glossy white circle around edge of cornea) due to fat deposits
- Decreased corneal sensitivity
- Development of presbycusis, progressive sensorineural hearing loss, affecting filtering of high-frequency sounds ("f," "ph," "s," "sh," "ch") from speech
- Decrease in number of touch receptors, reduced tactile sensitivity

FAST FACTS in a NUTSHELL

Changes to sensory organ function create safety risks for older adults. For example, older individuals may be unable to effectively hear warning sounds, read instructions and warnings on labels, and sense pressure that is threatening skin breakdown. It is important to identify these risks during the assessment and develop plans to minimize them.

ASSESSMENT CONSIDERATIONS

Prior to examining the patient, perform a gross inspection noting any weakness, tremor, paralysis, asymmetry, deformity, twitching, or other abnormalities.

Ask the patient about pain, tingling sensations, headaches, dizziness, sleep disturbances, numbness, blackouts, changes in mental function, vision and hearing problems, and other symptoms that could indicate neurologic disorders. If the patient admits to having any symptoms, ask for a detailed description, including onset, relationship to other events, effects on function, and efforts to manage them.

As the nervous system is complex and affects many areas of function, an organized approach to assessing this system is essential. Specific areas to assess include:

- *Speech and language:* Communication involves the use of symbols (language) and articulation by the motor apparatus (speech); therefore, the assessment will aid in revealing the nature of any communication problems that may be present. Specific problems to note are:
  - *Dysarthria:* This is a difficulty with articulation; the problem may be with motor control of the tongue, pharynx, lips, or a combination of these. Speech will be slurred, mumbled, or distorted but there will be correct use of words. Subtle dysarthria can be elicited by having the patient repeat the syllables la, la, la (to test motor control of the tongue), ga, ga, ga (to test the pharynx), and me, me, me (to test lip control). You can also have the patient repeat the phrase "Methodist Episcopal," which will reveal dysarthrias.
  - *Dysphasia:* This is impairment in the use of symbols. Paraphasia is a mild form involving the substitution of one word for another (e.g., calling a watch a clock). Dysphasias can have a receptive or expressive component, or both. To assess for receptive problems, ask the patient to follow commands, such as "point to your nose" or "pick up that pencil." With expressive dysphasia, the patient can understand and follow a direction properly, but not communicate the words.
- *Olfaction:* Cranial nerve I is the olfactory nerve. To test olfaction, use a substance with a distinct scent, such as coffee or rose, and ask the patient to identify the scent as you occlude each nostril separately. Identifying the exact scent is less important than the ability to determine that a scent is present. Keep in mind that there are nonneurological reasons for the loss of a sense of smell.
- *Visual acuity:* The most common method for testing visual acuity is the Snellen chart. If the patient wears glasses determine visual acuity with the glasses worn, testing one eye at a time. The most common cause of decreased visual acuity is presbyopia.

- *Visual field:* A gross determination of visual field can be derived by having the patient sit and positioning yourself approximately 3 feet away with your eyes level with the patient's eyes. Ask the patient to look directly at your eyes as you stretch your arm midway between you and the patient and point your

=== *FAST FACTS in a NUTSHELL*

You can use a newspaper to determine what level of type the patient is able to see (e.g., headlines only, small text). This may have more meaning to caregivers in understanding the patient's visual capacity than a Snellen chart reading.

finger up. As the patient and you continue to look directly at each other's eyes, gradually bring your finger into the peripheral field and ask the patient to indicate when he or she sees your finger. Systematically test all points along a 360° area in the visual field. Older adults often have reduced peripheral vision and will not see your finger at the same distance as you.

=== *FAST FACTS in a NUTSHELL*

Patients may display blind areas in their visual field. A blind area that accompanies glaucoma is known as scotoma. People who have had cerebrovascular accidents can have blindness in the same half of the visual field of both eyes; this condition is known as homonymous hemianopsia. Sometimes patients are unaware that they have these conditions until tested. Repeatedly bumping into objects or ignoring items placed in the same area of the visual field could give clues to the presence of these types of conditions.

- *Extraocular movements:* Cranial nerves III, IV, and VI (the oculomotor, trochlear, and abducens nerves) act in concert to control extraocular eye movements. A test of this function is to have the patient look straight ahead and, using your finger as a target, ask him or her to follow your finger as you move it to various horizontal and vertical locations. Normally, the eyes should move together with no jerking movement.

- *Pupil response to light:* The oculomotor nerve also controls the relationship of the lid to the pupil and the light reflex. To test this nerve's function, have the patient look straight ahead and bring in a flashlight from the side; constriction is the normal response. Also inspect the lids for drooping, ptosis, which is an abnormal finding.
- *Facial nerve:* Cranial nerve VII is the facial nerve that controls the muscles of facial expression. Inspect the patient's face for symmetry and for symmetrical movement when the patient talks or smiles. Asking the patient to smile, show his or her teeth by raising the lips, and tightly closing both eyes further tests this nerve.
- *Hearing:* Hearing loss can be conductive, in which case there is a problem in the passage of sound through the canal, ossicles of the middle ear, or the tympanic membrane; or sensorineural, in which case the problem is associated with the inner ear receptors or the nerve itself. Cranial nerve VIII, the vestibulocochlear nerve, is responsible for hearing and balance. A gross test of hearing can be done by going behind the patient and speaking in a whisper. If the patient cannot hear the whisper, gradually raise the volume of your voice until you are heard.

FAST FACTS in a NUTSHELL

Some patients compensate for hearing loss by lip reading. By going behind the patient and speaking to test hearing, you help avoid this and prevent missing a hearing deficit.

- *Gag reflex:* Cranial nerves IX (glossopharyngeal) and X (vagus) control the pharynx and palate. To test the function of these nerves, ask the patient to say "ah"; normally, the uvula should rise.
- *Shoulder movement:* Cranial nerve XI (cranial) supplies the sternomastoids and trapezius. To test its function, ask the patient to shrug his or her shoulders and note symmetry of movement. A lag of one side is abnormal.
- *Tongue movement:* The hypoglossal nerve, cranial nerve XII, controls the movement of the tongue. Ask the patient to stick out his or her tongue and move it from right to left several times. Note any deviation in movement.

- *Coordination:* Test the patient's coordination using point-to-point tests. Hold your finger out and ask the patient to touch his or her nose and then your finger. Move your finger to different positions and repeat. Test both arms. Normally there should be smoothness of movements. Also, test tandem walking by having the patient walk heel to toe. If necessary, hold the patient's hand for safety.
- *Reflexes:* Deep tendon reflexes typically are not tested during routine nursing assessments. Superficial reflexes can be tested by touching the cornea with a wisp of clean cotton; the normal response is for the eye to blink. Babinski's reflex (plantar response) is tested by stroking the sole of the foot; the normal response is for the toes to flex.
- *Sensation:* Ask the patient to close his or her eyes and touch various parts of the body with a wisp of cotton and gently with a pin. The patient should be able to sense and differentiate the sensations at various parts of the body.
- *Mental status:* Cognitive changes can indicate neurological disorders. A full discussion of mental status assessment and conditions is provided in Chapter 11.

CONDITIONS

Cataracts

Cataracts, the leading cause of low vision in the older population, are a loss of transparency of the lens due to a clouding of the lens or its capsule. Some degree of lens opacity occurs in all individuals as they age. Factors that contribute to the formation of cataracts include exposure of the eyes to sunlight, cigarette smoking, diabetes, high alcohol consumption, and eye injury.

Many people miss the symptoms of cataracts as they develop because in the early stage visual acuity is not affected. However, as opacification advances, the following symptoms occur:

- Distorted, blurred vision
- Difficulty with night vision
- Feeling like there is a film over the eye
- Sensitivity to glare and bright light

- Cloudy appearance to the pupil
- Yellow or yellow-brown discoloration of the lens due to nuclear sclerosis

Changes to the lens can cause some people to experience an improvement in near vision.

Due to the sensitivity to glare, it is beneficial for persons with cataracts to protect the eyes from bright light and glare by:

- Wearing sunglasses
- Using several soft sources of lighting or indirect lighting rather than large bright lights; avoid fluorescent lights
- Preventing direct sunlight from shining through windows with the use of blinds and sheer curtains

FAST FACTS in a NUTSHELL

Because older persons have more problems adjusting to contact lenses and special cataract glasses, the insertion of an intraocular lens during the cataract surgery is preferred. This is easier for patients than having to care for contact lenses and tends to result in less distortion of vision than glasses produce. Complications can occur with a lens implant, such as eye infection, loss of vitreous humor, and slipping of the implant.

Surgery is the only means of curing cataracts and the ophthalmologist will determine the appropriateness and timing of surgery for individuals. Cataract removal is a common outpatient surgery that tends to be well-tolerated by older adults. For older patients, intracapsular extraction, in which the lens and capsule are removed, is the surgical procedure of choice. With extracapsular extraction, which is a simple surgical procedure, the lens is removed and the posterior capsule is left in place. A common problem with extracapsular extraction is that a secondary membrane may form, requiring an additional procedure for discission of the membrane. Postoperatively patients can resume normal functions, avoiding strenuous activities.

Glaucoma

Glaucoma is a degenerative eye disease in which an increase in intraocular pressure due to a buildup of aqueous humor in the eye damages the optic nerve. The prevalence of glaucoma increases with age. The condition affects women more than men and tends to develop earlier in African American persons. Persons with an increased lens size, family history, iritis, allergy, and endocrine imbalance are at higher risk of developing glaucoma; the exact cause is unknown, however. Because they dilate the pupil, anticholinergic drugs can increase symptoms in person with this condition.

FAST FACTS in a NUTSHELL

Following cataracts, glaucoma is the second most common eye problem of older adults and the second leading cause of blindness for this age group.

Chronic Glaucoma (Open Angle)

Most cases of glaucoma are the chronic form. There is an insidious onset, causing people to be unaware that they are experiencing vision problems until the disease has progressed to an advanced stage. Symptoms include:

- Poor vision in dim lighting
- Increased sensitivity to glare
- Tired feeling in eyes
- Need to frequently change eyeglass prescription
- Headaches
- Impaired peripheral vision; as the condition progresses central vision is impaired
- Dilated pupil, cloudy appearance of cornea
- Perception of halos around lights

Both eyes are usually affected, although chronic glaucoma can affect a single eye.

Chronic glaucoma usually is managed with medications to reduce intraocular pressure and can include miotics, prostaglandins, beta-blockers, adrenergic agonists, and carbonic anhydrase inhibitors. In some cases surgery may be required, such as iridectomy, iridencleisis, cyclodialysis, and corneoscleral trephining.

Acute Glaucoma (Closed Angle)

A sudden blockage of the flow of aqueous humor causes this medical emergency that requires prompt attention to avoid blindness. Symptoms occur abruptly and include:

- Severe eye pain
- Headache
- Nausea, vomiting
- Blurred vision

The individual needs to be examined by an ophthalmologist who will conduct a visual field test (perimetry) and obtain a tonometry reading. Additional tests may be performed to differentiate open angle from closed angle glaucoma.

Treatment may include medications to reduce the formation of aqueous solution, such as carbonic anhydrase inhibitors and mannitol, or glycerin, which reduce fluid because of their ability to increase osmotic tension in the circulating blood. To prevent recurrence, an iridectomy may be performed after the acute attack.

Patients with glaucoma should not overuse or strain their eyes. Stimulants, mydriatics, and other medications that elevate the blood pressure can increase intraocular pressure and should be avoided in persons who have glaucoma.

FAST FACTS in a NUTSHELL

Patients with glaucoma need to be conscientious about the administration of their eye medications.

[**Clinical Snapshot**]

During his evaluation, Mr. G's intraocular pressure is found to have significantly increased. Concerned, the ophthalmologist is considering an increase in medication. The nurse questions Mr. G about his current routine of administering his eye drops. "Well," responds Mr. G, "because my fingers are so stiff with arthritis, I waste a lot of the drops when trying to put them in, and with them being so expensive, I just couldn't afford to keep doing that, so I stopped using them. I didn't notice any problem."

The lack of finger dexterity to use a dropper, the cost of the drugs, and the silent nature of the disease that causes him to be unaware of the changes occurring may be greater contributors to Mr. G's increase in intraocular pressure than a progression of disease. Helping him to obtain assistive devices to compensate for his stiff fingers or exploring the possibility of someone else instilling the drops for him, along with reinforcing the importance of regular administration of the drugs, could prove more beneficial than increasing the dose of the drugs.

MACULAR DEGENERATION

The most common cause of blindness in older adults is macular degeneration. With this condition there is damage or breakdown of the macula, resulting in a loss of central vision. Although it can result from injury or infection (exudative macular degeneration), the most common form, involutional macular degeneration, occurs due to the aging of the eye. Routine ophthalmic examination can detect macular degeneration and assist in early treatment that can prevent additional vision loss. This emphasizes the importance of encouraging and assisting older adults to have regular ophthalmic examinations.

Some types of macular degeneration are treated with laser therapy; unfortunately, the involutional form does not respond well to this treatment. Patients with this condition can be aided by the use of magnifying glasses, high-intensity reading lamps, and other aids.

Detached Retina

Retinal detachment occurs when there is a forward displacement of the retina from its normal position against the choroid. Symptoms vary depending on the extent of the detachment and can occur gradually or suddenly; they include:

- Perceiving spots moving across the eye
- Blurred vision
- Flashes of light
- Sensation that there is a coating over the eye
- Blank areas of vision that progress to complete loss of vision

Immediate attention is necessary to avoid the progression of symptoms and ultimate blindness. Initially, the use of an eye patch and bed rest are prescribed. In time, surgery to reattach the retina can be done.

FAST FACTS in a NUTSHELL

Several types of surgical techniques are used to treat detached retinas. To return the retina to its original attachment, electrodiathermy and cryosurgery can be performed. Scleral buckling and photocoagulation are procedures that are done to decrease the size of the vitreous space.

Patients need explanations, support, and reassurance throughout the treatment, as symptoms and the prescribed treatment can be frightening.

Hearing Deficits

Hearing loss is common in older adults and can result from a variety of factors, including:

- Exposure to loud noise (e.g., machinery, jets, loud music)
- Recurrent otitis media

- Trauma to the ear
- Ototoxic drugs (e.g., aspirin, ethacrynic acid, furosemide, indomethacin, erythromycin, streptomycin, neomycin, rauwolfia derivatives)
- Disease (e.g., diabetes mellitus, hypothyroidism, syphilis)
- Tumors
- Inner ear damage from vascular conditions or viral infections
- Otosclerosis (osseous growth leading to fixation of the foot plate of the stapes in the oval window of the cochlea)
- Cerumen impaction

Although common in late life, hearing deficits should not be assumed to be normal or irreversible; therefore, audiometric examination is needed to determine the cause and possible treatment.

FAST FACTS in a NUTSHELL

When hearing cannot be improved, interventions to help the person live safely and communicate effectively are necessary. It is not unusual for individuals with hearing loss to limit social contacts due to feeling self-conscious about their hearing deficits or to become angry and impatient at what they perceive to be the poor communication style of others whom they are unable to properly hear. These individuals should be assisted in obtaining hearing aids, if determined to be appropriate, and urged to request to have information provided in writing or repeated to ensure it is understood. Safety measures such as alarm systems that use blinking lights in addition to audible sounds can prove useful.

Hearing aids can benefit some persons with hearing deficits. Because not all hearing deficits can benefit from these aids, it is important that an otologist conduct an evaluation and recommend the best aid for the patient. The patient needs to understand that a period of adjustment is typically needed with a new hearing aid, and hearing will not be restored to its previous normal level. It is not uncommon for speech to sound distorted with the aid, and for reverberation and amplification of environmental sounds to cause annoyance. Patients should be instructed in the proper care of the aid, which includes:

- Turning the aid off or removing the battery when not wearing it
- Storing the aid in a padded, safe, dry container when not being worn
- Avoiding exposure of the aid to temperature extremes
- Cleaning the aid weekly and as needed by wiping it off and removing cerumen and other particles from the channel with a pipe cleaner or special pick device that may come with the aid
- Having several new batteries readily available

Transient Ischemic Attacks

A transient ischemic attack (TIA) is a neurological event arising from a reduction in cerebral circulation that can last from minutes to hours and cause symptoms such as:

- Aphasia
- Unilateral loss of vision
- Diplopia
- Hemiparesis
- Hemianesthesia
- Vertigo
- Nausea, vomiting, dysphagia

TIA can result from a reduction in cerebral circulation (e.g., when a person rises suddenly from a lying position or hyperextends or flexes the head), hypotension, or vasoconstriction from cigarette smoking and certain medications). Treatment includes correcting the underlying cause, anticoagulant therapy, and in some situations, vascular reconstruction. Symptoms typically subside within a day; however, there is concern as having a TIA increases the person's risk for a cerebrovascular accident (CVA).

Cerebrovascular Accidents

CVA is the severe, sudden decrease in cerebral circulation caused by either a thrombus or embolus or a hemorrhage from a ruptured vessel; a thrombus is the most common cause in older persons.

The incidence is higher among people with hypertension, atherosclerosis, diabetes mellitus, anemia, hypothyroidism, and those with a history of cigarette smoking and TIA.

═══ *FAST FACTS in a NUTSHELL*

CVAs are a major cause of disability and the third leading cause of death among older individuals.

The onset and type of symptoms can vary depending on the area of the brain involved. Common signs associated with CVA can include:

- Paralysis (usually hemiplegia)
- Hemianopsia
- Aphasia
- Lightheadedness, dizziness
- Drop attack (complete muscular flaccidity in lower extremities without alteration in consciousness)
- Change in level of consciousness
- Impaired memory and judgment

Prompt identification of signs and medical attention can prevent death and serious disability.

═══ *FAST FACTS in a NUTSHELL*

It is beneficial to understand the part of the brain affected, as function can vary depending on the hemisphere involved. With a left hemisphere lesion, there will be right hemiplegia; impaired ability to read, write, and speak; some impairment of comprehension; and slow, cautious movements; the person is aware of deficits and prestroke function tends to be more easily restored. Persons with right hemisphere lesions have no awareness of deficits, poor judgment, short attention span, an inability to transfer learning, more performance than comprehension problems, and are less likely to regain prestroke capabilities.

In the acute phase, the goals are to:

- Maintain an open airway
- Monitor neurological and vital signs
- Provide adequate hydration and nutrition
- Prevent complications (e.g., pressure ulcers, contractures, pneumonia, aspiration, corneal damage from eyes remaining open for an extended time)

As the patient's condition stabilizes, rehabilitative measures will be implemented. Although plans will be based on the patient's individual capacities and limitations, some general nursing measures include:

- Provide consistency of caregivers.
- Speak to the patient during caregiving activities. Explain procedures and activities in a clear, simple manner. Avoid shouting.
- Utilize a picture chart to aid communication.
- Place photographs and familiar objects in the patient's room. Include a calendar and clock.
- Provide positive feedback for progress. Remember, even minor actions can reflect a significant accomplishment for the patient.
- Show patience. Care activities may take longer and the patient may have periods of slow progress.
- Recognize that anger, depression, and other feelings may be expressed and offer support.
- Allow opportunities for the patient and his or her family to express feelings.
- Consult with physical and occupational therapists for specific exercises and aids that can benefit the patient.

Parkinson's Disease

Parkinson's disease is a progressive neurological condition that affects the ability of the central nervous system to control body movement. It results when the dopamine-producing neurons die or are damaged. The incidence increases with age, occurring most often after the fifth decade of life.

The onset of symptoms tends to be subtle, often beginning with a faint hand tremor that progresses over time and is reduced when the patient attempts a purposeful movement; a pill-rolling motion of the fingers may accompany this. As the disease progresses, other symptoms develop, such as:

- Muscle weakness and rigidity
- Slow, monotone speech
- Masklike facial expression
- Shuffling, rapid gait with forward leaning of trunk and lack of arm swing; inability to voluntarily stop walking
- Stooped posture
- Poor balance
- Increased appetite
- Difficulty swallowing, drooling
- Bradykinesia (slow movement)
- Urinary hesitancy, urgency
- Reduced interest in sex
- Disturbed sleep
- Emotional instability (depression, anxiety)
- Dementia, in some cases

FAST FACTS in a NUTSHELL

Levodopa, usually in combination with carbidopa, is prescribed for most people with Parkinson's disease to control symptoms. Several months of therapy may be needed before intended effects are achieved. Side effects could include nausea, vomiting, anorexia, lightheadedness, dyskinesia, and altered cognitive function.

Controlling symptoms, promoting maximum independence, and preventing complications are major goals of care. Nursing interventions can include:

- Reviewing the impact of the disease on activities of daily living and planning interventions according to deficits
- Administering medications and teaching the patient and/or caregivers about medications

- Maintaining joint mobility through range-of-motion exercises and joint massage
- Monitoring urine output for signs of retention
- Preparing family and caregivers for patient's emotional swings, which often accompany the disease; offering emotional support
- Respecting the patient's intellectual ability and offering intellectually stimulating activities
- Reducing stresses that can cause frustration and tension, which aggravate symptoms
- Monitoring status to identify increased risks for complications
- Ensuring patient is treated with respect and patience
- Consulting with physical and occupational therapists for strategies to maintain and promote function

Ongoing monitoring and assessment of the patient are important due to the progressive nature of the disease, which affects caregiving needs.

9

Integumentary System

The integumentary system serves important functions in terms of protection to the body, comfort, and self-image. Efforts to compensate for lines and wrinkles, maintain adequate skin moisture, and prevent skin injury and disease are among the challenges older adults face as they experience the effects of aging on this system.

Objectives

In this chapter you will learn to:

1. Identify age-related changes to the integumentary system
2. Describe components of the assessment of the integumentary system
3. Recognize the clinical signs and describe the care of older patients with:
   - Pruritus
   - Keratosis
   - Seborrheic keratosis
   - Pediculosis
   - Scabies
   - Pressure ulcers
   - Skin cancer

AGE-RELATED CHANGES

Changes to the skin, hair, and nails are quite noticeable reflections of the aging process. The impact of aging on the integumentary system is affected by a variety of factors, such as genetics, diet, exposure to ultraviolet light, hygienic practices, medications, and lifestyle behaviors. Common changes include:

- "Thinner," drier, more fragile skin due to flattening of the epidermal-dermal junction, reduced thickness and vascularity of dermis, reduced epidermal proliferation
- Reduced skin elasticity due to coarser collagen fibers and degeneration of elastin fibers
- Skin wrinkling, sagging, and lines
- Increased skin fragility
- Increased risk for skin infections due to reduced skin immune response
- Increased benign and malignant skin neoplasms
- Reduction in melanocytes
- Thinning; reduced growth; and graying of scalp, axillary, and pubic hair due to loss of pigment cells and atrophy and fibrosis of hair bulbs
- Thicker hair in nose and ears
- Slower growth of nails, increased brittleness of nails
- Reduced perspiration due to reduction in number and function of sweat glands

FAST FACTS in a NUTSHELL

Solar elastosis or photoaging is sun-induced damage and premature aging of the skin due to exposure to ultraviolet rays. The damage is especially high to fair-skinned persons. Avoiding excess exposure to ultraviolet rays and the use of sun-screening lotions when outdoors can reduce these effects and promote skin health.

Multiple concerns arise from these changes, the most obvious being the effects on body image. Skin that is wrinkling and sagging and hair that is graying and being lost heighten the reality of growing old. This can result in anxiety, depression, and social withdrawal. It also can cause people to spend considerable money on products and services that promise to reverse the effects of aging. Although engaging in activities that enhance appearance can have positive outcomes, caution is needed to prevent older adults from wasting money or subjecting themselves to harmful products and procedures. Also, the fragility of the skin increases the risk for skin tears, pressure ulcers, and other disruptions to skin integrity. Once skin integrity is compromised in older adults, healing takes longer and the risk for infection is high.

ASSESSMENT CONSIDERATIONS

Assessment of the integumentary system begins on first contact with the patient by noticing color, condition, care, and abnormalities of the skin, hair, and nails. Unusual findings in the integumentary system could be related to problems beyond this system. For example, unclean skin, hair, and nails can be due to altered cognition, depression, lack of home heating, pain, or limitations in movement. Skin rashes or discolorations can arise from medications, allergies, or disease processes. Likewise, skin breaks or sores can be due to falls, reduced sensations, or limited mobility.

FAST FACTS in a NUTSHELL

The general health and function of the individual should be considered when assessing unusual findings in the integumentary system, as disease processes and limitations in self-care abilities can be manifested through skin problems.

Ask the patient about symptoms that could indicate problems within this system, such as itching, dryness, burning, or unusual or recent hair loss. Review bathing and shampooing practices. Most older patients do not need daily baths or showers and can suffer increased skin dryness from them; daily partial baths with complete bathing only every several days or as needed usually can suffice.

An examination of the total body surface is the optimum way to assess this system. The particular aspects to note include:

- *Skin color:* Inspect the entire skin surface. It is best to use a nonfluorescent light, as fluorescent lights can make it more difficult to detect fine rashes and lesions. Identify areas that differ from the rest of the skin color, noting location, color, size, onset, and related symptoms. Findings could include:

- *Redness:* Pressure or inflammation can cause a specific area of redness. Generalized redness can result from fever, alcohol intake, and exposure to extreme environmental temperatures.
- *Bluish discoloration:* This occurs due to a reduction in hemoglobin associated with hypoxia and most frequently is apparent on the lips, nail beds, and oral mucosa. Causes include cardiac or respiratory disease, anxiety, or a cold environment.
- *Irregular brown patches, similar to freckles:* These commonly occur on parts of the body exposed to sunlight but also could be associated with Addison's disease, hyperthyroidism, and other conditions.
- *Yellow discoloration of the sclera, mucous membranes, and skin:* This usually is caused by jaundice. With chronic renal disease there can be a yellow discoloration of the skin but the sclera and mucous membranes are not affected.
- *Paleness:* A variety of conditions can cause the skin to lose color or become pale, such as albinism, anemia, shock, and fatigue.
- *Moisture:* Note excessively oily, dry, or sweaty areas.

FAST FACTS in a NUTSHELL

Some Black-skinned individuals may have skin that is dry and flaky. This is a condition known as ash and is a normal finding. Moisturizer can aid in lubricating the skin and reducing ash.

- *Temperature, texture, turgor:* Using the back of your hands, determine temperature, comparing one side of body to the other. Note the smoothness or roughness. Decreased elasticity causes poor skin turgor to be a common finding in older adults; assessing at the forehead and sternum are the best sites to assess turgor, as they lose elasticity less than other parts.
- *Lesions:* Describe any lesions by their:
  - Distribution: generalized, specific area
  - Type (see Table 9.1)

TABLE 9.1 Types of Skin Lesions

Macule: small spot or discoloration, nonpalpable, texture similar to surrounding skin

Papule: a discoloration, 1/2 cm or less in diameter with firm palpable elevation

Plaque: a group of papules

Vesicle: fluid-containing lesion less than 1/2 cm in diameter that with a palpable elevation

Pustule: a lesion containing purulent fluid, of variable size with palpable elevation

Bulla: a fluid-filled lesion more than 1/2 cm in diameter with a palpable elevation

Wheal: a red or white palpable elevation that may occur in variable sizes

Nodule: a lesion 1/2 to 1 cm in diameter with firm palpable elevation; the skin may or may not be discolored

Tumor: a lesion exceeding 1 cm in diameter with firm palpable elevation; the skin may or may not be discolored

Fissure: a groove in the skin

Ulcer: an open depression in the skin of variable sizes

- *Configuration:* clustered, in a circle (annular), in a straight line, separate
- *Nails:* Examine and palpate the fingernails and toenails. Press on several nails to test for blanching. Normally the pink color should return to the nail bed; poor return can be associated with anemia or circulatory insufficiency. Brown, red, or white hairline lines under the nail can be caused by trauma, although some can appear for no apparent cause. Brown or black pigmentation of the nails can be a normal finding among black-skinned persons. Transverse ridges along the nail bed (furrowing or Beau's lines) can be present due to injury to the nail or severe systemic illness. Fungal infections of the toenail (onychomycosis) will appear as dry, scaly-looking material under the nail. Splitting of the nail at the distal portion (onycholysis) should be noted.
- *Hair:* Note grooming and condition. If present, ask about hair loss, flaking of the scalp, unusual hair growth, and other problems. Examine the scalp for lesions, discolorations, lice, and tender areas.

FAST FACTS in a NUTSHELL

Tender, red areas of the hairline along the temple accompanied by pulsations of the superficial temporal arteries can indicate giant cell arteritis. This finding should be referred for evaluation.

CONDITIONS

Pruritus

The age-related dryness that accompanies aging heightens the risk for itching to arise, known as pruritus. Although this problem is often caused by excessive bathing and dry heat, it can also be associated with diseases such as diabetes, hyperthyroidism, cancer, liver disease, pernicious anemia, uremia, and scabies, as well as some psychiatric conditions. With having more fragile skin, older adults can traumatize their skin by the itching; therefore, preventing and promptly addressing this problem are essential. The underlying cause should be corrected. In some circumstances, antihistamines and topical steroids and zinc oxide may be used to control the itching. Moisturizing lotions and bath oils can aid in preventing this problem.

Keratosis

Small, light gray or reddish-brown colored lesions with a rough texture are keratoses—also called solar or actinic keratoses. They typically occur on exposed areas of the skin. They can be removed through surgical excision, cryosurgery (freezing with liquid nitrogen), phytodynamic therapy, or topical agents (e.g., 5-fluorouracil, imiquimod, diclofenac). Although benign, keratotic lesions can be precancerous and require close observations for changes.

Seborrheic Keratosis

Of the many skin growths that occur with age, seborrheic keratosis is the most common. Occurring on various parts of the body, these yellow-brown, greasy-looking growths can be as small as a speck or as large as the size of a quarter, flat or wart-like. These growths are benign, however, older adults may be interested in having them removed for cosmetic purposes. It is important that seborrheic keratosis be evaluated and differentiated from precancerous lesions.

Pediculosis

Lice infestations can affect older adults, particularly those living in nursing homes, assisted living communities, and other settings in which they reside in close contact with others. They are spread through direct contact with the infected individual or items used by that individual (e.g., linens, combs, clothing). The easiest lice to detect are pubic lice (pediculosis pubis) that appear as small gray flecks on pubic hairs. Head lice (pediculosis capitis) can appear as white specks in the hair accompanied by itching; weeping, crusty areas can develop on the scalp as the condition continues. Body lice (pediculosis corporis) are difficult to detect; small red, macular lesions and severe itching are major signs. These infestations are highly contagious and require prompt treatment. Removal of the nits with a fine comb, the use of pediculicides, and discarding contaminated items or washing them in very hot water are part of the treatment. Assessment of persons in close contact with the patient should be done, as they may also require treatment.

Scabies

Another highly contagious infestation is scabies, caused by itch mites. The major sign is severe itching that usually is worse at night. The flexor surface of the wrist, digital web spaces, axilla, nipples,

FAST FACTS in a NUTSHELL

Persons infected with pediculosis or scabies need to have their bedding, clothing, and towels decontaminated. The Centers for Disease Control and Prevention recommends decontamination of these items by washing in hot water and drying in a hot dryer, dry-cleaning, or sealing in a plastic bag for at least 72 hours.

and genitalia are the most common sites. Inspection of the affected area reveals a whitish-gray linear pattern with a dark dot at the end; lesions can be macular, papular, vesicular, or nodular. Treatment consists of the application of a scabicide to the entire body and decontamination of clothing and linens.

Pressure Ulcers

A pressure ulcer is an impairment to skin integrity and/or underlying tissue caused by pressure or the combination of pressure and shear. The heels and sacrum are the sites where pressure ulcers most frequently develop; the ears, elbows, coccyx, and ischium are other common sites. Older adults are not only at high risk for the development of pressure ulcers, but can suffer threats to quality of life and general health status as a result of them. A variety of factors contribute to the development of pressure ulcers in older adults, such as:

- Increased fragility of skin
- Immobility (both for the bedbound and chairbound person)
- Malnourishment
- Impaired cognition
- Incontinence
- Extended time on an operating room table during surgery

The high risk for impaired skin integrity reinforces the need to assess the patient's skin status and risk at admission, readmission, and periodically thereafter. Halogen or natural lighting is superior to fluorescent lights to detect skin color changes, particularly in

FAST FACTS in a NUTSHELL

Individuals with darkly pigmented skin are more likely to have Stage I pressure ulcers inadequately detected and experience more severe tissue injury in Stages II to IV pressure ulcers than Whites (VanGildner et al., 2009). This requires that nurses understand the normal skin color of patients with dark skin pigmentation, look for subtle color changes, compare skin over bony prominences to that of surrounding area, and assess for skin temperature changes and sensitivity.

dark-skinned persons. A variety of tools can be used to identify pressure ulcer risk, such as the Braden Scale (Bergstrom, Allman, & Carlson, 1994), Norton scale (Norton, McLaren, & Exton-Smith, 1962), and the Pressure Sore Status Tool (PSST) (Bates-Jensen, 1996).

For a patient newly admitted to a facility who is at high risk for pressure ulcer development, it is useful to assess the skin status after 1 hour, as this could be sufficient time for skin breakdown to occur in some patients. If there is no evidence of pressure after 1 hour, wait 2 hours and check again. If the patient is able to remain in the same position for 2 hours without evidence of pressure, an every 2-hour turning and repositioning schedule can be planned; however, if pressure is noted in a lesser time frame, hourly turning and repositioning should be planned.

If a pressure ulcer is present it needs to be accurately staged. The National Pressure Ulcer Advisory Panel has developed categories and stages which are considered the standard for assessing pressure ulcers (see Table 9.2). Regular descriptions of the pressure ulcer's characteristics need to be noted, including the:

- Location, measurement, depth, and stage of the ulcer
- Presence or absence of exudate, slough, or necrosis
- Evidence of granulation
- Status of surrounding skin

In addition to an individualized turning and repositioning schedule, there are additional interventions that could prove beneficial, such as:

- Addressing causative or contributing factors (e.g., improving nutrition, using improved urine containment measures, increasing mobility)
- Using alternating pressure mattresses, heel protectors, and other devices to redistribute pressure
- Consulting with dietician as to nutritional approaches
- Developing and following an individualized bathing schedule; using moisturizers; avoiding hot water and harsh soaps, which can dry the skin
- Following prescribed treatment measures (e.g., special dressings, debriding agents)

TABLE 9.2 National Pressure Ulcer Advisory Panel (NPUAP)Pressure Ulcer Stages/Categories

International NPUAP-EPUAP Pressure Ulcer Definition

A pressure ulcer is localized injury to the skin and/or underlying tissue usually over a bony prominence, as a result of pressure, or pressure in combination with shear. A number of contributing or confounding factors are also associated with pressure ulcers; the significance of these factors is yet to be elucidated.

Pressure Ulcer Stages/Categories

Category/Stage I: Nonblanchable erythema
Intact skin with nonblanchable redness of a localized area usually over a bony prominence. Darkly pigmented skin may not have visible blanching; its color may differ from the surrounding area. The area may be painful, firm, soft, warmer, or cooler as compared to adjacent tissue. Category I may be difficult to detect in individuals with dark skin tones. May indicate "at-risk" persons.

Category/Stage II: Partial thickness
Partial thickness loss of dermis presenting as a shallow open ulcer with a red pink wound bed, without slough. May also present as an intact or open/ruptured serum-filled or sero-sanginous-filled blister. Presents as a shiny or dry shallow ulcer without slough or bruising.* This category should not be used to describe skin tears, tape burns, incontinence associated dermatitis, maceration or excoriation.

Category/Stage III: Full thickness skin loss
Full thickness tissue loss. Subcutaneous fat may be visible but bone, tendon, or muscle is *not* exposed. Slough may be present but does not obscure the depth of tissue loss. *May* include undermining and tunneling. The depth of a Category/Stage III pressure ulcer varies by anatomical location. The bridge of the nose, ear, occiput, and malleolus do not have (adipose) subcutaneous tissue and Category/Stage III ulcers can be shallow. In contrast, areas of significant adiposity can develop extremely deep Category/Stage III pressure ulcers. Bone/tendon is not visible or directly palpable.

Category/Stage IV: Full thickness tissue loss
Full thickness tissue loss with exposed bone, tendon, or muscle. Slough or eschar may be present. Often includes undermining and tunneling. The depth of a Category/Stage IV pressure ulcer varies by anatomical location. The bridge of the nose, ear, occiput, and malleolus do not have (adipose) subcutaneous tissue and these ulcers can be shallow. Category/Stage IV ulcers can extend into muscle and/or supporting structures (e.g., fascia, tendon or joint capsule), making osteomyelitis or osteitis likely to occur. Exposed bone/muscle is visible or directly palpable.

*Bruising indicates deep tissue injury.

(continued)

TABLE 9.2 National Pressure Ulcer Advisory Panel (NPUAP)Pressure Ulcer Stages/Categories (*continued*)

Additional Categories/Stages for the USA

Unstageable/Unclassified: Full thickness skin or tissue loss – depth unknown

Full thickness tissue loss in which actual depth of the ulcer is completely obscured by slough (yellow, tan, gray, green, or brown) and/or eschar (tan, brown, or black) in the wound bed. Until enough slough and/or eschar are removed to expose the base of the wound, the true depth cannot be determined but it will be either a Category/Stage III or IV. Stable (dry, adherent, intact without erythema or fluctuance) eschar on the heels serves as "the body's natural (biological) cover" and should not be removed.

Suspected Deep Tissue Injury – depth unknown

Purple or maroon localized area of discolored intact skin or blood-filled blister due to damage of underlying soft tissue from pressure and/or shear. The area may be preceded by tissue that is painful, firm, mushy, boggy, warmer or cooler as compared to adjacent tissue. Deep tissue injury may be difficult to detect in individuals with dark skin tones. Evolution may include a thin blister over a dark wound bed. The wound may further evolve and become covered by thin eschar. Evolution may be rapid, exposing additional layers of tissue even with optimal treatment.

From the National Pressure Ulcer Advisory Panel, 2009, Washington, DC. Reprinted with permission.

- Preventing, identifying, and taking prompt actions to correct complications, such as pain, cellulitis, osteomyelitis, depression
- Monitoring and documenting pressure ulcer status and healing progress

Skin Cancer

The most common skin cancers among older adults are:

- *Basal cell carcinoma:* The most common form of skin cancer, these are small, dome-shaped elevations covered with small blood vessels that resemble flesh-colored moles; sometimes the surface is dark. They can occur anywhere on the body, although the face is a common site. In addition to aging, exposure to ultraviolet and therapeutic sources of radiation increases the risk for this cancer. They are slow growing and rarely metastasize; however, if left untreated, they can spread and invade bone and other tissues.

- *Squamous cell carcinoma:* This cancer develops on the squamous cells that are located on the skin surface, the lining of the hollow organs of the body, and the passages of the respiratory and digestive tracts. It typically appears as firm, skin-colored or red nodules. Exposure to sunlight is the most common factor contributing to this cancer, although exposure to radiation, arsenic, and hydrocarbons are factors in some cases. Metastasis is common.

- *Melanoma:* Melanomas have been increasing in incidence in the United States; the incidence rises with age. They have a tendency to metastasize, which contributes to them being highly deadly if not diagnosed and treated early. There are several types of melanomas, each of which has a slightly different presentation:

  - *Superficial spreading melanoma:* The most common form that can occur anywhere on the body. This appears as a variably pigmented plaque with an irregular border.

  - *Lentigo maligna melanoma:* This is a flat lesion that can be black, brown, white, or red. Sun-exposed areas of the body are the most common sites for it. As it grows, the lesion becomes increasingly irregularly pigmented.

  - *Nodular melanoma:* Occurring anywhere on the body, this is a dark-pigmented papule that grows in size over time.

Any suspicious lesion should be evaluated and biopsied. Typically, melanomas are surgically removed, along with surrounding tissue and subcutaneous fat. It is the depth, not type, that affects the prognosis.

FAST FACTS in a NUTSHELL

Many older adults may go for an extended period without having a full-body examination that could detect lesions; therefore, they should be advised to independently inspect their bodies for new lesions and existing moles that have changed size or color and to bring their findings to the attention of their medical provider.

10

Endocrine System

> The body contains a system of glands that secrete hormones that help to maintain homeostasis. Hormones, the body's chemical messengers, regulate important functions, such as metabolism, sleep, mood, tissue repair, reproduction, and growth and development. Aging causes a decline in hormone production that produces effects that are highly noticeable and common among older individuals, including increased weight, fatigue, cold extremities, sleep disturbances, reduced immunity, decreased libido, and depression. In late life, diabetes, hyperthyroidism, and hypothyroidism are particular concerns associated with this system and threats to health, function, and quality of life. Efforts to promote the health of this system and effectively manage disorders related to glandular function are common challenges in geriatric care.

Objectives

In this chapter you will learn to:

1. Identify age-related changes to the endocrine system
2. Describe components of the assessment of the endocrine system

3. Recognize the clinical signs and describe the care of older patients with:
   - Diabetes mellitus
   - Hypothyroidism
   - Hyperthyroidism

AGE-RELATED CHANGES

A variety of changes in the glands and their secretion of hormones occur with age, affecting a wide range of bodily functions; these include:

- Atrophy and reduced activity of the thyroid gland, which results in:
  - Slower metabolism
  - Decreased secretion of thyrotropin
  - Reduced radioactive iodine uptake
  - Reduction in total serum iodine released, although protein-bound iodine levels in the blood are unchanged
  - Reduction in triiodothyronine (T3)
- Decrease in the size of the pituitary gland, which results in reductions in:
  - ACTH
  - Thyroid-stimulating hormone (TSH)
  - Follicle-stimulating hormone
  - Luteinizing hormone
  - Luteotropic hormone
  - Testosterone
  - Estrogen
  - Progesterone
- Decrease in secretory activity of the adrenal gland (related to reduced secretion of ACTH, which regulates this gland), affecting reductions in secretions of:
  - Aldosterone
  - Glucocorticoids
  - 17-ketosteroid
  - Progesterone
  - Androgen
  - Estrogen
- Delayed and insufficient release of insulin by beta cells of pancreas

FAST FACTS in a NUTSHELL

Older adults have a high prevalence of endocrine and metabolic dysfunction as compared to other age groups. Hypothyroidism, osteoporosis, diabetes mellitus, adrenal insufficiency, hypopituitarism, various forms of hypogonadism, and endocrine malignancies occur more frequently in late life. Evaluation of diagnostic tests differs, as does treatment of these conditions.

ASSESSMENT CONSIDERATIONS

Symptoms and family history related to endocrine system diseases should be reviewed. During the general assessment there are a variety of complaints and signs that could be associated with disorders of the endocrine system, such as:

- Heat or cold intolerance
- Sweating or flushing
- Change in skin texture, excessive dryness of skin and hair
- Weakness
- Weight changes
- Diarrhea, constipation
- Increase or decrease in usual blood pressure or pulse rate
- Sleep disturbances
- Erectile dysfunction
- Enlargement of male breasts
- Polyuria
- Polydipsia
- Polyuria
- Loss or increase in body hair
- Slow wound healing
- Decreased ability to manage stress

Ask about the presence of these symptoms and, if present, explore the history of onset, pattern, and effects on daily life.

   Physical examination can reveal problems suggestive of endocrine disorders; note:

- Exophthalmos
- Visible enlargement of the thyroid gland

- Depigmentation of skin. This often occurs on the face, neck, extremities, and mucous membranes
- Thick, brittle fingernails
- Areas of abnormal hair growth

A blood sample can show abnormalities consistent with various endocrine problems, such as:

- Fasting blood glucose
- Glycosylated hemoglobin (HbA1c)
- TSH
- T3
- T4
- Serum calcium
- Serum phosphate
- Cortisol
- Aldosterone

Glucose tolerance testing can be done if there are indications of specific problems. In addition, urine samples can be tested for glucose, ketones, and microalbumin.

When endocrine problems are suspected, further evaluation is warranted. This could include magnetic resonance imaging (MRI), computed tomography (CT), thyroid scan, and radioactive iodine uptake test (RAI).

CONDITIONS

Diabetes Mellitus

The growing prevalence of obesity, less active lifestyles, and improved diagnostic measures have added to the age-related changes that contribute to a growing prevalence of type 2 diabetes in the aging population. Early diagnosis is often difficult because symptoms can be attributed to other chronic conditions. Primary symptoms associated with hyperglycemia include:

- Polyuria
- Polydipsia (although older adults often have impaired thirst mechanisms)

===== *FAST FACTS in a NUTSHELL*

In persons over age 65 years of age, 27% have diabetes and 50% are prediabetic based on fasting glucose or hemoglobin A1c levels. (Centers for Disease Control and Prevention, 2013).

- Polyphagia
- Weight loss
- Fatigue, weakness, drowsiness after meals
- Dry eyes and mouth
- Glycosuria

===== *FAST FACTS in a NUTSHELL*

Because the renal threshold for glucose increases with age, older adults with diabetes may not demonstrate glycosuria.

Later symptoms could include:

- Slow wound healing
- Increased infections
- Blurred vision
- Foul-smelling breath
- Altered mental status

According to the American Diabetes Association (2010), any one of the following could be a diagnostic indicator for diabetes:

- Random blood glucose $\geq$200 mg/dL and primary symptoms of hyperglycemia
- Glycosylated hemoglobin (HbA1c) $\geq$6.5%
- Fasting blood sugar (8 hour fast) $\geq$126/dL
- 2-Hour blood glucose value during oral glucose tolerance test $\geq$200 mg/dL with glucose load of 75 g

Interventions for older persons with diabetes are basically the same as those for any age group.

FAST FACTS in a NUTSHELL

If the individual is malnourished or recently experienced an illness or period of inactivity, it is important to share this with the medical provider, as these situations can be a factor in glucose intolerance.

FAST FACTS in a NUTSHELL

A thorough nutritional assessment is essential for older persons with diabetes. Included would be a review of weight history, usual eating patterns, supplements and medications used, food-drug and food-supplement interactions, caloric intake and needs, food budget, meal preparation, ethnic/cultural dietary preferences and restrictions, psychosocial factors affecting nutritional intake, knowledge of proper nutrition and diabetes management, and attitude about changing dietary habits. The active participation of the team nutritionist is valuable to developing an optimum plan.

Strict glycemic control in persons of advanced age and those with multiple comorbidities can result in greater harm than benefit, so the impact of treatments must be evaluated carefully (Steinman & Hanlon, 2010). Patient education is essential and can be challenging for older individuals who are overwhelmed or anxious about their diagnosis. Offering emotional support is important to laying the foundation for effective patient education. Topics to include in the teaching plan include:

- Realities about the disease
- Medications: administration, dosage, precautions, etc. (see Table 10.1)
- Diet
- Weight management
- Signs of hypoglycemia and hyperglycemia and related actions to take
- Foot care (see Table 10.2)
- Signs of complications

TABLE 10.1 Hypoglycemic Agents

Drug Group	Examples	Nursing Considerations
Sulfonylurea drugs	Glibenclamide Glipizide Gliclazide Glimepiride	Sulfonylurea tablets should be taken a half-hour before meals. It is recommended that the drug be started at a low dose, about half of the usual adult dosage, and gradually increased if required. Main side effects are hypoglycemia and weight gain. Glibenclamide use in older persons carries a risk for severe hypoglycemia, believed to be related to delayed clearance of the active metabolites of this drug.
Alpha-glucosidase inhibitor	Acarbose	Flatulence and other gastrointestinal disturbances can occur, which can be minimized by starting with a smaller dose and gradually increasing the dosage if necessary.
Short-acting insulinotropic	Repaglinide	This is a nonsulfonylurea that acts by augmenting endogenous insulin secretion from the pancreas in response to a meal; can be taken with meals. Hypoglycemia can occur but the risk is lower than with the sulfonylureas. Contraindicated in persons with liver or renal disease. Insulin sensitizers: thiazolidinediones
Rosiglitazone Pioglitazone		Insulin sensitizers used alone or in combination with sulfonylureas, metformin, or insulin. Side effects can include weight gain, edema, pulmonary edema, and congestive heart failure, so monitoring for symptoms of these conditions is necessary.
Biguanide	Metformin	Used with people who have no abnormality in renal, cardiac, or respiratory functions; can produce abdominal discomfort, anorexia, bloating and diarrhea as side effects; not recommended for people over age 80 due to increased risk for metabolic acidosis.

========= *FAST FACTS in a NUTSHELL*

Basal-bolus insulin may be used in the management of diabetes, as it simulates natural insulin delivery and is associated with less hypoglycemia. Basically, the basal is the basic insulin dose that is given daily and the bolus is the dose given at mealtimes to cover the specific food intake. Bolus insulins include Regular, Aspart (Novolog), Glulisine (Apidra), and Lispro (Humalog). Basal insulins include NPH, Detemir (Levemir), and Glargine (Lantus).

Older adults who need to self-administer insulin may have specific challenges due to problems in handling the syringe, such as arthritic joints or administering the correct dosage due to vision or cognitive impairments. Likewise, they may have difficulty testing blood glucose levels. Their competency to perform these tasks needs to be evaluated before they are sent home to independently manage these activities. It may be necessary to instruct a family member or neighbor who can assist with these activities. In addition, a variety of assistive products are available that can aid patients in managing their condition; these include syringe magnifiers, audio blood glucose meters, and insulin pens. Information on these resources can be obtained through occupational therapists and the Academy of Nutrition and Dietetics' Diabetes Care and Education Practice Group (www.dce.org).

========= *FAST FACTS in a NUTSHELL*

Older adults with diabetes and their caregivers need to advise medical practitioners of the diagnosis of diabetes when new medications are prescribed. Hypoglycemia can occur when beta-blockers, salicylates, warfarin, sulfonamides, tricyclic anti-depressants, and alcohol are used by older persons who are diabetic. In addition, older adults should be cautioned not to use over-the-counter medications without discussing this with their medical provider or a pharmacist to ensure the drugs do not interact with ones being used or affect glycemic levels.

Patient education is important. People with diabetes and their caregivers should be taught about:

- The proper use and storage of medications
- Recognition of hypo- and hyperglycemia.
- The importance of not substituting medications; reinforce that all insulins or oral antidiabetic drugs are not interchangeable
- The need to examine injection sites regularly if insulin is used as local redness, swelling, pain, and nodule development at the injection site can indicate insulin allergy
- The need to notify their health care provider if they develop fever; prolonged diarrhea or vomiting; altered thyroid function; or heart, kidney, or liver disease as these could alter antidiabetic drug requirements
- Not using a new medication without discussing it with their health care provider first

Ongoing monitoring is important, which would include testing of:
- Hemoglobin A1c: Usually done quarterly, this measures the amount of glycosylated hemoglobin in the blood and is helpful in evaluating the effectiveness of disease control. Hemoglobin A1c provides an average of the patient's blood glucose control over a 6- to 12-week period; the normal range is between 4% and 6%. For persons with diabetes, the goal is a HbA1c below 7%.

=============== *FAST FACTS in a NUTSHELL*

Antidiabetic medications can interact with many other drugs and cause serious effects. For example, the effects of antidiabetic drugs can be:

- *Increased by alcohol, oral anticoagulants, cimetidine, isoniazid, phenylbutazone, ranitidine, sulfinpyrazone, and large doses of salicylates*
- *Decreased by chlorpromazine, cortisone-like drugs, furosemide, phenytoin, thiazide diuretics, thyroid preparations, and cough and cold medications*

- Triglycerides: The American Diabetes Association recommends that people with diabetes maintain their triglyceride levels below 150 mg/dL.

Identifying complications is also part of the monitoring activity. Older adults are at higher risk of developing complications from their diabetes than younger adults. In addition, recognition of these complications in an early stage can be difficult due to altered presentation of symptoms. For example, hypoglycemia may present with behavior problems, convulsions, somnolence, confusion, disorientation, poor sleep patterns, nocturnal headache, slurred speech, and unconsciousness rather than the classic symptoms of tachycardia, restlessness, perspiration, and anxiety. Numbness, weak pulse, infection, and gangrene can arise due to peripheral vascular disease, which is a common complication in older persons with diabetes; this reinforces the importance of good foot care in older persons with diabetes (see Table 10.2). Additional complications that are at high risk to older adults with diabetes include urinary tract infection, cognitive impairment, neuropathies, carpal tunnel syndrome, postural hypotension, coronary artery disease, and cerebral arteriosclerosis.

FAST FACTS in a NUTSHELL

Persons with type 2 diabetes have twice the risk of developing dementia. (Strachan, Reynolds, Marioni, & Price, 2011)

Living with diabetes can be a challenge for older adults. It can require changing dietary and lifestyle habits that have been practiced for decades. Freedom may be limited and extra burdens imposed on already burdened lives by the need to check blood glucose levels, administer medications, and visit a medical provider more often. Regular support and reinforcement of care needs, as well as evaluation of continued competency to meet them, are part of the ongoing care of these individuals. A variety of free educational resources

TABLE 10.2 Foot Care for Persons With Diabetes

Diabetes can affect nerves that can signal excessive temperatures, pressure, and pain. As a result, injuries to the feet can occur more easily and take longer to be recognized. Good foot care practices are essential to foot health. The following offers foot care guidelines to persons with diabetes.

Daily Foot Care
- Wash feet in warm water with a mild soap or soak the feet. Dry gently with a towel, especially between the toes.
- Examine the feet, noting dry skin, cracks, lesions, cuts, blisters, bruises, or changes in color. If eyesight is not good, arrange for a family member or caregiver to inspect the feet at least once a week.
- Apply lotion to soften the skin. Do not apply lotion between the toes.

Toenail Care
- Use nail clippers to cut nails straight across. Do not cut into corners to round the toenails or cut a nail shorter than the edge of the toe.
- Gently file sharp edges with an emery board.
- Do not cut your own nails if there is a problem with poor vision, unsteady hands, or ability to reach the toes.
- Have a podiatrist care for nails if they are thick, cracked, or split.

Caring for Corns and Calluses
- After washing feet, gently rub corns or calluses with a soft towel.
- Do not peel off, cut, or use drugstore remedies to remove corns and calluses.
- Wear properly fitting shoes.

General Considerations
- Do not use hot water bottles, heating pads, or hot soaks on feet.
- Wear shoes that fit well and are comfortable. Avoid going barefoot.
- Inspect the inside of shoes for stones and other foreign material before putting them on.
- Wear clean socks that fit well and do not constrict.
- Notify the physician if there is any cut or sore on the foot that doesn't improve within a day, or if there is any sign of infection, numbness, or discoloration.

that can aid in helping persons with diabetes live a full, high-quality life are available from the National Diabetes Education Program at www.ndep.nih.gov.

Hypothyroidism

Hypothyroidism, the subnormal concentration of thyroid hormone in tissues, increases in prevalence with age and is more common in women. There are two types:

- *Primary hypothyroidism:* This is caused by a disease process that destroys the thyroid gland, and is characterized by low free T4 or free T4 index with an elevated TSH level.
- *Secondary hypothyroidism:* Insufficient pituitary secretion of thyroid-stimulating hormone (TSH) is the major cause of this type. It is characterized by low free T4 or free T4 index and low TSH.

Symptoms of hypothyroidism are easily confused with other geriatric conditions and include:

- Weight gain
- Dry skin, coarse hair
- Cold intolerance
- Fatigue, lethargy, weakness
- Constipation
- Puffy face
- Periorbital or peripheral edema
- Myalgia, paresthesia, ataxia
- Depression, apathy

Treatment consists of thyroid hormone replacement therapy, using a synthetic T4 such as synthroid or thyroixine. Usually a low dosage is prescribed, as rapid elevation of thyroid levels could exacerbate symptomatic coronary artery disease. Close monitoring is important when therapy is started to evaluate the effects of the specific dosage level.

Hyperthyroidism

Although less prevalent than hypothyroidism, the condition in which the thyroid gland secretes excess amounts of thyroid hormones, hyperthyroidism, does occur among older persons. A potential cause of this is iodine-induced hyperthyroidism, often related to the use of the cardiac drug amiodarone, which contains iodine that deposits in tissue and delivers iodine to the circulation over very long periods of time. Overdosage of thyroid hormone replacement therapy also can be a contributing factor.

Symptoms of hyperthyroidism include:

- Diaphoresis
- Tachycardia
- Nervousness
- Hypertension
- Palpitations
- Tremor
- Insomnia
- Confusion
- Heat intolerance
- Increased hunger
- Proximal muscle weakness
- Hyperreflexia
- Exopthamos
- Diarrhea

FAST FACTS in a NUTSHELL

Hyperthyroidism-related diarrhea may not be present if the older person has had a history of chronic constipation. Rather than diarrhea, the person may develop regular bowel movements.

Diagnostic tests include evaluation of T4 and free T4, TSH, and increased uptake of radionuclide thyroid scans. T3 levels may be unreliable if the person has a poor nutritional status, as that will have reduced the T3 level. Therefore, the disease-related elevation could bring the T3 into a normal range.

The underlying cause will determine the treatment approach and could include antithyroid medication, radioactive iodine, or surgery.

II

Mental Status

Mental status encompasses mood and cognitive function. Although there is no normal decline in mental status that occurs with age, there can be a wide range of intellectual abilities and emotional states found among older adults. This is a feature of differences in genetic makeup, general health status, lifestyle choices, activity level, education, and experiences. Further, if mental health implies the ability to make appropriate decisions, engage in activities of interest, and derive a satisfaction from life, there can be differences that prevent a stereotype from being developed.

There are challenges in late life that can affect mental health, such as widowhood, reduced income, caregiver stress, new health problems, relocation, and retirement. Health issues and the shrinking availability of a support system can increase the burden of managing these challenges and affect mental health. Nurses must view older adults holistically to understand the factors impacting mental status and provide appropriate interventions.

Objectives

In this chapter you will learn to:

1. Identify age-related changes to mental status
2. Describe age-related changes to memory, intelligence, learning ability, attention, and personality
3. Describe components of a mental status assessment
4. Recognize the clinical signs and describe the care of older patients with:
   - Delirium
   - Dementia
   - Depression
   - Substance abuse

AGE-RELATED CHANGES

FAST FACTS in a NUTSHELL

Cognitive function includes memory, thinking, perception, learning and thinking.

Findings regarding mental health in late life need to be put in perspective of the individual's normal mental status throughout life. Neither the intellectually sharp 80-year-old executive who continues to competently manage her corporation nor the anxious 75-year-old who is unable to complete a basic health questionnaire represent the norm for all older adults. Bright elders may have demonstrated high intellectual function their entire lives while intellectually limited older persons may have always performed at a basic level. An understanding of lifelong intellectual and emotional function is essential to providing insight into the individual's norm and any changes that may have occurred due to pathological processes. Aging affects cognition in the following ways:

- *Memory:* Throughout the years research has offered various, and sometimes conflicting, views on memory and aging. It now is thought that there is some decline in both long-term and short-term memory; this may be due to the large amount of information that is stored in that memory. Memory can be affected by age-related changes that slow processing, education, personality, learning habits, sociocultural background, physical and mental health status, and task demands. Relevant, interesting, and positive information or emotional stimuli results in memory recall and recognition that is at least equal to that of younger adults (Blanchard-Fields & Kalinauskas, 2009).

- *Intelligence:* Basic (crystallized) intelligence involving the ability to use past learning and experiences for problem solving is unchanged. There is believed to be some decline in fluid intelligence that is responsible for processing new information, spatial perception, and creative capacities.
- *Learning:* Basic learning ability is unchanged, although there can be a tendency to rely on past experience to problem-solve rather than utilize new techniques, and more factors (e.g., sensory deficits) can interfere with learning. Changes in intensity and duration of physiologic arousal with age can cause difficulties in changing old responses to acquire new information. In the early phase of learning older adults may not perform as well as younger persons; however, after a delayed early phase the differences are minimal. Perceptual motor tasks become more difficult.
- *Attention span:* Older adults are more easily distracted by stimuli and irrelevant information.

Personality, morale, and attitude normally are consistent through the lifespan, although health conditions and lifestyle challenges can cause some changes.

ASSESSMENT CONSIDERATIONS

Insight into mental status can be gained upon first introduction and observation of the individual. Observations to note include:

- *Grooming and dress:* Poor hygienic and grooming practices and inappropriate clothing and makeup could offer clues to cognitive or mood disorders.

- *Facial expression:* Pain, fear, anger, depression, and other feelings could be reflected through expressions.
- *Movement:* Repetitive movements, hand wringing, tongue rolling, hyper- or hypoactivity can be indicators of mental health issues.
- *Level of consciousness:* Drifting off to sleep and demonstrating difficulty or excessive slowness in responses are abnormalities to note.
- *Speech:* Problems can be revealed by the tone, rate, and content of speech.

Specific questions during the interview can surface mental health problems, even in individuals who otherwise appear to have no problems. Examples of questions include:

- How would you describe your mental condition?
- Are you feeling depressed, sad, nervous, fearful, or moody?
- Have you noticed any changes or problems with your thinking, memory, concentration, ability to focus? Do you ever think you are losing your mental abilities? If so, describe this.
- How often to you socialize with others? Has there been any change in this?
- How is your appetite? Has there been any recent change in it?
- Do you have trouble falling or staying asleep? If so, when did this start and what do you do about it?
- Do you use any medications, herbs, or alcoholic beverage to relax or affect your mood or mental function? What medications do you use? (List all medications, including when, where, and why ordered.)
- Do you ever hear voices or noises that other people don't? See things that other people don't?
- Do you look forward to each day?
- What brings you pleasure and purpose?
- Have you ever been hospitalized or treated for depression, anxiety, or any other emotional or mental problem? If so, describe this.

In addition to responses that could indicate alterations in mood or cognition, unusual tone, body language, or behaviors should be noted.

========================= *FAST FACTS in a NUTSHELL*

There are several evidence-based tools that can be used to test cognitive function, including the Short Portable Mental Status Questionnaire (Pfeiffer, 1975), the Philadelphia Geriatric Center Mental Status Questionnaire (Fishback, 1977), Mini-Mental Status (Folstein et al. 1975), Symptoms Check List 90 (Derogatis et al., 1974), General Health Questionnaire (Goldberg, 1972), OARS (Duke University, 1978), and, specifically for depression, the Zung Self-Rating Depression Scale (Zung, 1965).

There are a variety of reliable, validated tools that can be used for the mental status evaluation, and you should become familiar with the tool your organization uses and adhere to the policy and procedure for its use. Typical components of cognitive testing include:

- *Orientation:* Ask the person to state his name, where he is (e.g., doctor's office, nursing home), the city, state, date, time of day, and season.
- *Memory:* As you initiate the assessment, tell the person you are going to give three words (e.g., unrelated words such as clock, door, bread) for her to remember, state the words, and ask her to repeat the words. Midway through the assessment ask the person to state the words that she was asked to remember; repeat at the end of the assessment, also.
- *Three-stage command:* Instruct the person to perform three simple acts, such as pick up the piece of paper, fold it in half, and hand it to you.
- *Judgment:* Offer a situation to problem solve (e.g., "What would you do if you saw smoke coming from the next room?") or present a saying (e.g., "People in glass houses shouldn't throw stones") and ask the person to describe its meaning.
- *Calculation:* Ask the person to count backwards from 100 by 5s. If known intellectual or educational limitations are present, ask the person to count backwards from 20 by 2s. (Counting 5 increments backward is sufficient.)

FAST FACTS in a NUTSHELL

Catastrophic reactions can occur during the assessment if the person with dementia becomes overwhelmed at the challenges presented.

[Clinical Snapshot]

The nurse is assessing Mr. K, a nursing home resident who has Alzheimer's disease, and during the mental status component of the assessment asks Mr. K what type of place they are in. Mr. K. looks somewhat puzzled and responds, "Is it my daughter's house? No, a hotel? What is this place? Why are you keeping me here?" With that, Mr. K becomes very agitated, stands, and paces around the room. His reaction is known as a catastrophic reaction and occurs when persons with dementia become overwhelmed by the challenges presented and begin to display behaviors such as anger, crying, or withdrawal. The best approach would be for the nurse to temporarily stop the assessment and help to calm Mr. K.

All abnormal or unusual findings should be documented in as much detail as possible.

Laboratory evaluation of blood (e.g., complete blood count, electrolytes, glucose, sedimentation rate, serologic test for syphilis, vitamin levels) and urine may be ordered, as physiological imbalances and diseases can cause mental status alternations. If specific problems are suspected, other diagnostic tests may ordered, such as electroencephalography, computed tomography, magnetic resonance imaging, and positron emission tomography scan.

CONDITIONS

Delirium

Delirium is a syndrome characterized by a sudden (hours or days) impairment in cognitive function, including:

• Disorientation to time and place
• Impairment of recent memory (e.g., the person may not be able to recall that he is in a hospital)

- Disorganized thinking; rambling, incoherent conversation
- Illusions, hallucinations; misperceptions of familiar people and objects
- Inattentiveness, easy distractibility

Level of consciousness is disturbed and psychomotor activity can fluctuate from hyperactivity (agitation, restlessness, increased activity) to hypoactivity (slow movement, unresponsiveness). Symptoms can fluctuate throughout the day. Sleep-wake cycle is affected also.

FAST FACTS in a NUTSHELL

There is a high prevalence of delirium among hospitalized older adults, which is often persistent after discharge and can result in increased disability and mortality (Dasgupta & Hillier, 2010).

Virtually anything that disrupts the body's balance can cause delirium; this can include:

- Dehydration
- Malnutrition
- Electrolyte imbalances
- Hyper- or hypothermia
- Hyper- or hypoglycemia
- Hypothyroidism
- Hypotension
- Adverse drug reactions
- Congestive heart failure
- Infections
- Surgery
- Decreased cardiac function
- Decreased respiratory function, hypoxia
- CNS disturbances
- Pain
- Emotional stress

Patients with new acute conditions or who are hospitalized are at particularly high risk for developing a delirium. Deliriums can develop in persons with dementias; understanding the individual

FAST FACTS in a NUTSHELL

The high risk for developing delirium and its serious conse-quences reinforce the importance of knowing the older adult's normal mental status, regularly assessing and monitoring mental status, and identifying changes early.

with dementia's normal mental function and behavior can assist in recognizing changes indicative of a delirium.

Any change in cognition, behavior, or level of consciousness demands evaluation. The condition is reversible with early treat-ment of the underlying cause. In addition to supporting the treat-ment plan to address the cause, nursing interventions include:

- Limiting the stimuli and number of people with whom the patient has contact
- Providing frequent orientation, explanations, reminders, and support
- Placing a clock and calendar in the patient's room
- Ensuring the patient wears prescribed eyeglasses and hearing aids
- Placing familiar objects in the environment
- Providing adequate lighting to avoid misperceptions of the en-vironment, avoiding bright lights
- Ensuring basic needs (nutrition, toileting, bathing, grooming, ambulating) are met, pain is controlled, and medications are administered
- Monitoring vital signs, intake and output, neurologic status
- Evaluating the environment for potential safety hazards (e.g., unlocked windows, solutions left in the room, clutter)
- Checking on the patient often to prevent injury
- Providing comfort and relaxation measures (e.g., massage, soft music, aromatherapy)
- Encouraging and assisting family and significant others to spend time with the patient, offering them support and infor-mation as appropriate

Dementia

Dementia is a broad medical term that encompasses brain disorders in which there is a gradual irreversible decline in cognitive function, affecting memory, orientation, judgment, reasoning, attention, language, and problem solving. There is no change in level of consciousness. As the disease progresses, behavior, personality, and self-care ability are affected. There are several types of dementia, with Alzheimer's disease being the most common (Table 11.1).

TABLE 11.1 Types of Dementia

- *Alzheimer's disease,* the most common type of dementia, is characterized by the presence of neuritic plaques and neurofibrillary tangles in the cortex. It can be years before brain changes cause symptoms, which develop gradually and progress at different rates among affected persons.
- *Vascular dementia* is a rapidly progressing dementia caused by small cerebral infarctions that result in localized or diffuse damage to the brain. It is associated with risk factors such as smoking, hypertension, hyperlipidemia, inactivity, and a history of stroke or cardiovascular disease.
- *Frontotemporal dementia* is characterized by neuronal atrophy affecting the frontal lobes of the brain. In the early stage, behavioral changes are noted more than cognitive ones. Abstract thinking and speech and language skills are initially impaired more so than memory. Pick's disease is the most common form of frontotemporal dementia.
- *Lewy body dementia* involves subcortical pathology and the presence of Lewy body substance in the cerebral cortex. Fluctuations in mental status are common. There is a higher incidence among people who have a family history of dementia.
- *Creutzfeldt-Jacob disease* is an extremely rare dementia that is believed to originate from a slow virus. Symptoms appear and progress rapidly, and tend to be more diverse than Alzheimer's disease. Psychotic behavior, heightened emotional lability, memory impairment, loss of muscular function, muscle spasms, seizures, and visual disturbances are classic symptoms. Death typically occurs within 1 year of diagnosis.
- *Others:* Dementia can result from trauma, toxins, alcoholism, AIDS, and Parkinson's disease.

FAST FACTS in a NUTSHELL

An estimated 5.2 million Americans of all ages have Alzheimer's disease, which includes an estimated 5 million people age 65 and older and approximately 200,000 individuals younger than age 65 who have younger-onset Alzheimer's. (Alzheimer's Association, 2013)

Improved diagnostic techniques have aided in differentiating the various types of dementia, although identifying and differentiating dementia in an early stage remains challenging. Diagnosis typically is made through the mental status examination in which cognitive function is assessed and the history of symptoms are determined, indicating impairments in at least two of the following impairments (McKhann et al., 2011):

- Ability to acquire and remember new information
- Reasoning, judgment, or management of complex tasks
- Ability to recognize common objects
- Language function
- Mood, personality or behavior

In addition, there will be a decline in function and interference with the ability to engage in routine activities. It is important that a delirium or psychiatric disorder be ruled out. Accurate diagnosis enables treatments to be implemented that could correct causes and allow care to be planned in relation to the anticipated course of the specific dementia.

Although there are some unique features to each type of dementia, and their progression can occur at different rates, there are some general characteristics associated with mild, moderate, and advanced stages of the disease:

- *Mild:*
  - Routine activities become more difficult to perform
  - Judgment, decision-making, and problem-solving abilities are impaired
  - There is less engagement in work and social activities

- Processing spatial and visual information is more challenging
- Personality and mood changes may be present
- Person may be aware of changes and become depressed or withdrawn
- *Moderate:*
  - Worsening of cognitive function, increased confusion occurs
  - Disorientation to time and place is present
  - Mood changes may be more apparent, delusions and hallucinations may be present
- *Advanced:*
  - All areas of cognition are impaired
  - There is difficulty recognizing familiar people and places
  - Sleep-wake cycle is altered
  - Physical function and mobility are impaired, there is increased need for assistance with all activities of daily living
  - Significant personality changes occur
  - Behavioral problems are displayed

Care of persons with dementia includes actions to address those needs that they can no longer fulfill on their own; nursing actions include:

- Ensure safety
  - Have the person wear some form of identification that includes name and who to contact if the person is lost.
  - Have a recent photograph of the person available to aid in identifying and locating the person in the event of wandering away from the premises.
  - Maintain a stable, consistent environment.
  - Place alarms on doors to signal when a person tries to exit.
  - Use protective gates to limit wandering.
  - Monitor nutritional status and intake and output.
  - Administer medications and/or instruct caregivers in safe medication administration. Monitor the effects and potential side effects and adverse reactions to medications.
  - Store medications, cleaning supplies, pesticides, and other inedible substances that could be accidentally ingested in locked cabinets or inaccessible locations.

- Ensure the environment is free from clutter or obstacles in main walking paths.
- Cover outlets, motors, and other items in which fingers or foreign objects could be inserted and harmed.
- Ensure windows are locked or have nonremovable screens.
- Observe and monitor the actions of the person.
- Utilize alternatives to physical and chemical restraints.
- Promote orientation
  - Clarify misperceptions and use verbal cues to keep the person oriented.
  - Have calendars and clocks in the environment.
  - Keep photographs of relatives and friends in the environment labeled with names.
- Control stimuli
  - Control noise exposure. If possible, place the person in a room that does not have much hall traffic or noise.
  - Maintain a stable environmental temperature.
  - In health care facilities, consistently assign the same caregivers to the person.
  - Avoid harsh, bright lights.

FAST FACTS in a NUTSHELL

Sundowner syndrome can occur in persons with dementia and is characterized by agitation, disorientation, restlessness, wandering, and a general worsening of behavior as evening approaches (after the sun goes down). To aid in reducing the occurrence, maintain a stable environmental temperature, ensure basic needs are met, encourage daytime activity, provide orientation, and prevent pronounced transitions from light to dark by turning on lights before evening and using nightlights. Also, ensure the person is comfortable and has regular contact with others.

- Promote independent function
  - Obtain physical and occupational therapy consults and follow recommendations.
  - Adhere to routines in activities and schedules.
  - Limit choices the person has to make.

- Identify situations that trigger negative behaviors and try to avoid them.
- Assist with bathing, allowing the person to perform as much of the activity as possible.
- Put toothpaste on the brush and leave it on the sink.
- Lay out clothing and guide the person through the steps of dressing, one step at a time.
- Establish and adhere to an individualized toileting schedule.
- Offer easy-to-eat foods (e.g., finger foods, soft foods, foods that do not require cutting).
- Provide positive feedback.
- Facilitate communication
  - Use a relaxed approach.
  - Speak to the person in an adult voice, avoiding "baby talk" or a condescending tone.
  - Use simple sentences that contain only one idea.
  - Use simple, one-stage commands rather than offering multiple steps together.
  - If the person has difficulty understanding, try substituting alternative words for the ones used (e.g., if the person cannot understand, "Do you want to go to the activity room?" try asking "Would you like to go down the hall and listen to the music?")
  - Supplement verbal comments with visual cues as possible.
  - Allow ample time for the person to process and respond.
  - Avoid sarcasm or subtle humor.
  - Do not, and ensure others do not, mock or shame the person for incorrect word choices or incoherent verbalizations.
  - Observe nonverbal expressions and behaviors and attempt to interpret their meaning.
  - Be aware of your body language and facial expressions.

FAST FACTS in a NUTSHELL

As the dementia progresses and the person's capacities decline, it is important to ensure the person is treated with respect and that the preferences he or she has expressed through advance directives are honored.

- Provide support to family
  - Assess the family's knowledge and readiness to learn. (They may need assistance in working through their feelings before they can hear information presented.)
  - Educate the family about the disease, care, environmental modifications that may be helpful, and resources they can access for information and support.
  - Refer to legal and financial professionals for planning as needed.
  - Convey understanding of the burden they are carrying, demonstrate patience with their reactions, and provide support.
  - Encourage family to arrange periods of respite from their caregiving functions.

Depression

Although there are many factors that contribute to its occurrence, depression is not a normal outcome of aging. When it occurs, depression requires comprehensive evaluation to identify the cause and determine the appropriate treatment. Neglecting to treat this disorder can significantly threaten the quality of life and general health of the older adult.

According to the *Diagnostic and Statistical Manual of Mental Disorders (DSM-5)* a person has depression if there is no medical or physiological reason for the symptoms (e.g., hypothyroidism, neurological disorders, diabetes, adverse drug reaction), symptoms are not related to bereavement, and the person demonstrates either a depressed mood or loss of interest or pleasure and at least five of the following symptoms during a 2-week period of time:

- Depressed mood most of the day, nearly every day, as indicated by either subjective report (e.g., feels sad or empty) or observation made by others (e.g., appears tearful).
- Markedly diminished interest or pleasure in all, or almost all, activities most of the day, nearly every day.
- Significant weight loss when not dieting or weight gain (e.g., a change of more than 5 lbs of body weight in a month), or decrease or increase in appetite nearly every day.
- Insomnia or hypersomnia nearly every day.
- Psychomotor agitation or retardation nearly every day.

- Fatigue or loss of energy nearly every day.
- Feelings of worthlessness or excessive or inappropriate guilt nearly every day.
- Diminished ability to think or concentrate, or indecisiveness, nearly every day.
- Recurrent thoughts of death (not just fear of dying), recurrent suicidal ideation without a specific plan, or a suicide attempt or a specific plan for committing suicide.

FAST FACTS in a NUTSHELL

As many as 25% of older adults have depressive symptoms that do not meet the DSM criteria for depression, although the symptoms are significant and demand treatment. This has been categorized as minor depressive disorder if at least two depressive symptoms have been present for more than 2 weeks and the individual does not have a history of major depression. Common symptoms include are fatigue, insomnia, poor appetite, trouble concentrating, feelings of worthlessness, and recurrent thoughts of death.

Older adults may display depression differently from younger adults. For example, older adults are more likely to show cognitive changes, apathy, and physical complaints than affective symptoms that may characteristically present in younger persons.

FAST FACTS in a NUTSHELL

Some older individuals may display some impairment in cognitive function as a result of poor dietary intake and sleep disturbances related to being depressed. This is known as pseudodementia and can be mistaken as dementia to those unfamiliar with the usual function of these patients. This reinforces the importance of obtaining a good history to aid in identifying causes of the cognitive impairment seen and ensuring the underlying depression is properly treated. Asking family members of these individuals about recent changes in behavior and function and possible factors that precipitated them can also prove beneficial in differentiating dementia from pseudodementia.

When indications of depression are present, a thorough assessment is essential. An easy to administer screening tool that is widely used for assessing depression in older adults is the *Geriatric Depression Scale-Short Form (GDS-SF)*, which is available for free download from www.stanford.edu/~yesavage/GDS.html. It consists of 15 questions and can be completed in less than 10 minutes. Another short, quick assessment is the *Patient Health Questionnaire (PHQ-2)*, a two-question screening tool that is found to be particularly useful in assisted living communities and community settings (Watson et al., 2009). The two questions are simple: (1) asking the person if during the past 2 weeks (or month) he or she has felt down, depressed, or hopeless, and (2) felt little interest or pleasure in doing things. If a positive response is given to either of these questions, additional assessment is needed with a more formal depression tool.

FAST FACTS in a NUTSHELL

Lower rates of diagnosed depression are found in older African Americans, Asian Americans, and Native Americans. This is believed to be due more to missed diagnosis or misdiagnosis rather than an actual lower incidence (Harvath and McKenzie, 2012). Language barriers, lack of trust in the provider, and cultural attitudes about depression being inappropriate can be among the reasons depression is not reported by these individuals. Nurses should be particularly observant of atypical signs that could indicate depression (e.g., noncompliance with treatment plans, inattention to self-care, unusual carelessness or risk taking) and explore for depression as the cause.

When indications of depression are present, potential medical or pharmacologic causes that could contribute to the symptoms must be identified (Tables 11.2 and 11.3). As older adults commonly have chronic conditions and are prescribed many medications, these factors can be associated with depressive symptoms. In addition, life situations that could have contributed to depression need to be explored and addressed, such as recent loss of a loved one, relocation, new diagnosis, retirement, or financial challenges. Identifying potential factors that contribute to the depression is essential to developing an effective plan of care.

TABLE 11.2 Medical-Related Causes of Depression

- Cardiovascular conditions: congestive heart failure, angina, myocardial infarction
- Respiratory conditions: chronic obstructive pulmonary disease, lung cancer, pneumonia
- Gastrointestinal conditions: irritable bowel syndrome, malignancy, hepatitis
- Genitourinary conditions: urinary incontinence, urinary tract infection
- Musculoskeletal conditions: arthritis
- Neurologic conditions: cerebrovascular accident, transient ischemic attack, dementia, Parkinson's disease, normal pressure hydrocephalus, intracranial tumor
- Endocrine conditions: diabetes mellitus, hypothyroidism, hyperthyroidism, Cushing's disease, Addison's disease
- Metabolic conditions: acid-base imbalance, dehydration, uremia, abnormal levels of glucose, sodium, potassium, or calcium
- Other: pain, vitamin deficiencies, pernicious anemia, cancer

---

The cause, type, and severity of the depression determines the treatment. Treatment can include:

- *Antidepressant therapy:* Among the most popular drugs used to treat depression are:
  - Selective serotonin reuptake inhibitors (SSRIs): citalopram (Celexa), escitalopram (Lexapro), fluvoxamine (Luvox), paroxetine (Paxil), sertraline (Zoloft)
  - Cyclic compounds: amitriptyline HCl (Elavil, Amitril), amoxapine (Ascendin), desipramine HCl (Norpramine, Pertofrane), imipramine pamoate (Trofanil), nortriptyline HCl (Aventyl, Pamelor)
- *Electroconvulsant therapy (ECT):* This is used primarily for severe depressions, when antidepressant medications are ineffective. ECT is contraindicated for persons with serious cardiac disease and increased intracranial pressure.
- *Exercise:* Physical exercise has been shown to improve mood and reduce symptoms.
- *Psychosocial interventions:* For older adults with normal cognitive function, reminiscence, psychodynamic, and cognitive behavioral therapies have been shown to reduce depression.

TABLE 11.3 Medications That Can Cause Depression

- Analgesics: codeine, indomethacin, meperidine, propoxphene
- Antihypertensives and cardiovascular agents: clonidine, digitalis, hydralazine, methyldopa, reserpine
- Antiparkinsonian agents: levodopa
- Steroids: corticosteroids, estrogen
- Other: barbiturates, benzodiazepines, cimetidine, fluphenazine, levothyroxine sodium, varenicline

---

Nurses play an important role in developing and implementing an individualized plan that integrates the recommendations of all disciplines involved. Nursing interventions that can assist the older adult who has depression include:

- Monitor for status. The depressed person may not consume adequate food and fluid, obtain sufficient sleep, engage in hygienic practices, have regular bowel elimination, and be sufficiently active to prevent complications. Ensure basic needs are being met and provide assistance as needed.
- Observe for suicidal thoughts and acts. Suicide is a significant risk for depressed older adults. In addition to blatant acts, such as shooting or overdosing, subtle acts to end one's life may be attempted, such as omitting necessary medications, consuming excessive amounts of alcohol, ceasing to eat, or driving carelessly. Clues to suicidal thinking can include the person making a will, getting affairs in order, withdrawing from close relationships, and making funeral and burial plans. Any evidence of suicidal thinking or acts requires prompt psychiatric referral.
- Ensure contributing factors have been addressed (e.g., medications causing depressive symptoms have been changed, financial aid has been sought, malnutrition has been corrected).
- Encourage the expression of feelings. Allow and encourage the person to express guilt, anger, or any other feeling. Ensure caregivers and family members do not minimize the person's feelings or make judgments (e.g., "You shouldn't feel this way," "You have so much to be thankful for").
- Maximize opportunities for the person to make decisions and exercise control over his or her activities.

- Provide relaxation measures, such as music therapy, massage, diversional activities.
- Support and monitor the antidepressant therapy.
  - Ensure the correct dose is being administered.
  - Educate the person and caregivers about the medications, dosage, potential side effects, and adverse effects. Prepare them for the fact that several weeks of therapy may be needed before mood improvement occurs.
  - Review other prescription and over-the-counter drugs for potential interactions; if present, consult with physician about medication change.
  - Prepare the person for potential side effects, such as dry mouth, urinary retention, weight gain, photosensitivity, and drowsiness.
  - Observe for side effects and take action to prevent complications related to them.
- Ensure that follow-up care has been arranged, the person understands the plan, and has the ability to continue accessing care (e.g., financial ability, transportation).
- Refer the person and, as needed, family members to local support groups.

=== *FAST FACTS in a NUTSHELL*

Regardless of how minor the act may seem, acknowledge the person's efforts to take action to engage in self-care, participate in activities, and express feelings. This feedback can reinforce positive behaviors, encourage the person to adhere to the plan of care, and offer hope that progress is being made.

SUBSTANCE ABUSE

As the baby boomers reach old age, they are bringing an increased number of people with a history of alcohol and drug abuse into geriatric care circles. Substance abuse and dependency can go unnoticed because many providers do not consider these to be problems of older adults, and sometimes their manifestations can be mistaken as related to common geriatric conditions. Undetected, these problems can not only delay the correction of harmful behaviors, but also increase the risk for injuries and complications that can threaten the quality and quantity of life for older adults.

Alcohol is the most commonly abused substance in older adults; most older alcoholics have consumed alcohol heavily throughout their lives. Many chronic alcohol abusers have experienced the ill effects of this problem prior to reaching old age. Those who consumed alcohol regularly in younger years without adverse effects may find that consuming the same amount of alcohol in advanced years produces ill consequences.

Detecting alcoholism in older adults can be challenging. Rather than the boisterous, disruptive person who passes out at the bar, an older alcoholic can be the quiet widow who begins sipping brandy in the afternoon or the grandfather who consumes a six-pack of beer while working on a project in his garage. The first clue that there is a problem with alcoholism could be symptoms related to complications from alcohol abuse, such as altered cognition, malnutrition, depression, injuries, social isolation, hypertension, irregular heartbeat, heart failure, chronic infections, gastritis, magnesium deficiencies, pancreatitis, hepatitis, or cirrhosis. Questions about alcohol consumption should be included in the routine assessment. Concern for the presence of alcoholism should arise if the person:

- Drinks a fifth of whiskey or its equivalent in beer and wine daily
- Has a blood alcohol level >150 mg/100 mL
- Experiences blackouts
- Has convulsions, hallucinations, tremors, or delirium tremens (DTs) when abstaining from alcohol
- Refuses to cease drinking when advised to do so by a medical professional or when drinking-related problems are known to exist

FAST FACTS in a NUTSHELL

Although less common than alcohol use, illicit drug use can be present among older adults. In fact, we may be experiencing growing numbers of substance users in late life among the boomers who have had a history of marijuana and other drug use. Like alcohol use, questions about illicit drug use should be part of every assessment.

The type and severity of abuse and dependency determine the treatment plan. Treatment options could include detoxification, counseling, psychotherapy, cognitive behavioral therapy, pharmacologic treatment options (e.g., synthetic narcotic agonists), and community-based groups such as Alcoholics Anonymous and Narcotics Anonymous. These individuals and their families need to be educated about the risks associated with continued substance abuse and supported as they face the challenges of changing their behaviors.

Special Considerations in Geriatric Care

12

Spirituality

With the increasing prevalence of physical and mental health conditions with age, it is easy to overlook spiritual needs; however, the relationship between spirituality and general well-being is great in late life. Regardless of age, people have basic spiritual needs that include love, meaning and purpose, hope, forgiveness, gratitude, the expression of faith, and transcendence. In fact, some of these needs may take on greater significance for older adults, in light of the growing risk and prevalence of chronic conditions and the heightened awareness of the finiteness of life. Awareness that a spiritual self exists separate from the physical body enables older adults to find meaning, purpose, and satisfaction in the presence of illness, losses, and declining function. Helping older individuals to achieve that awareness and fulfill spiritual needs are essential components of holistic geriatric nursing care.

Objectives

In this chapter you will learn to:

1. Differentiate spirituality from religion
2. Identify basic spiritual needs
3. Outline questions to ask in assessing spiritual needs

4. Describe the general beliefs and practices of major religions
5. List signs of spiritual distress
6. Describe general actions to assist with spiritual needs

SPIRITUALITY VERSUS RELIGION

Every human being is a complex integration of body, mind, and spirit. To provide holistic care nurses need to be concerned with all of these aspects of the individual. Spirituality is not the same as religion, although religion can be part of a person's expression of spirituality.

FAST FACTS in a NUTSHELL

Spirituality refers to the essence of our being that transcends us as individuals and connects us to God or another higher power and other living organisms. The nature of spirituality is like the air we breathe: unseen, pervasive, boundless, and essential to life. Religion refers to a structure of symbols and rules created by humans with which we choose to identify and whose rituals we practice.

SPIRITUAL NEEDS

Spiritual needs encompass those aspects of one's life beyond the physical being that bring comfort, purpose, and peace to one's existence. These can consist of:

- *Loving and being loved:* Older adults, regardless of their ability to give physical gifts or perform physical tasks for others, are able to demonstrate unconditional love to others. In turn, they can receive love regardless of their condition or status.
- *Experiencing a life of meaning and purpose:* Most people feel a sense of wholeness when they sense that there is a reason to face each day. In late life, disease and disability can reduce the opportunities for purposeful activities; however, putting one's current life in perspective of the total life lived can aid the older adult in achieving a sense of integrity.

=== *FAST FACTS in a NUTSHELL*

One of the development tasks of late life is to achieve a sense of integrity by reviewing one's life and seeing the contributions and purpose of one's total life. Guiding the older adult through life review is one means to assist an older individual with this activity.

- *Having hope:* Anticipation of something in the future offers peace and comfort. That which is hoped for by the older adult can vary from recovery from an illness to making a long-desired trip to looking forward to eternal life in heaven.
- *Forgiving and being forgiven:* It is the rare individual who achieves old age without having done a wrong and causing hurt to another. For some, the cloud of the guilt associated with these acts is a tremendous burden. Asking for forgiveness can afford spiritual and emotional peace, as well as bring some comfort to the wronged person. Forgiving others also lifts burdens and can assist in re-establishing harmonious relationships with significant others in one's life.

=== *FAST FACTS in a NUTSHELL*

Forgiveness of oneself is significantly important to older individuals. Even when forgiveness is offered from others, some individuals continue to carry guilt and shame over past actions. Helping them to accept forgiveness and understand that mistakes are part of the human condition can aid in moving them toward self-forgiveness.

- *Offering thanks:* Declining health, retirement, reduced income, the death of loved ones, and the need to relocate are among the challenges faced by many older adults that can cause them to question what they have to be thankful for. They may need help in identifying the positive aspects of their lives and the value of the life experiences they have had.
- *Practicing one's faith:* A person's religious and spiritual beliefs can be expressed through prayer, worship, rituals, scripture

reading, and celebration of specific holy days. For the person of faith who has engaged in such practices, the disruption or inability to express their faith can be distressful.

- *Transcendence:* Transcendence implies the connection with something greater than one's physical world. For some people, this is an afterlife; anticipating this new life can aid in coping with the challenges faced by one's current life situation.

ASSESSMENT CONSIDERATIONS

A comprehensive assessment includes a review of spiritual needs. Insight into the patient's spiritual needs first can be gained by a review of the intake admission form for indications of the person's religion. The fact that a patient has stated that he or she is of a certain religion, agnostic, or atheistic hardly offers complete insight into spiritual needs, but it could aid in predicting some needs and preferences that can guide areas to explore during the assessment. Likewise, visible signs of faith practices, such as the wearing of religious articles or symbols, can offer insights. Specific questions that could be asked include:

- Do you practice a specific faith or religion? How important is this to your daily life? How do you practice it?
- Are you involved with a church, temple, or faith community? If so, what is it and would you like for them to visit you?
- Are there religious practices that are important to you that we can help you to engage in?
- Do you read the Bible or other religious text? Do you need assistance in reading it now?
- Is there anything about your faith, or religious or spiritual beliefs, that is causing you distress or discomfort now? If so, please describe it.
- What offers you meaning and purpose?
- Is there anything we can do to help you with your spiritual needs?
- Are there any dietary, activity, or other restrictions or practices related to your faith that we need to be aware of? (See Table 12.1, Religions and Their Practices That May Need to Be Considered in Caregiving.)
- Do you have any spiritual concerns or anything related to this that you'd like to discuss?

TABLE 12.1 Major Religions and Their Practices That May Need to Be Considered in Caregiving

PROTESTANTISM: Believe in Jesus Christ as Savior

- *Assemblies of God (Pentecostal):* Believe in divine healing through prayer and laying on of hands; communion provided by clergy; pray for God's intervention in healing; may abstain from tobacco, alcohol, and illegal drugs
- *Baptist* (more than two dozen different groups in the United States): Scripture reading important, as Bible viewed as word of God; may believe illness is God's will and respond passively to care; communion provided by clergy; some believe in healing power of laying on of hands; may abstain from tobacco, alcohol, and illegal drugs
- *Episcopal (Anglican):* Fasting not required, although some Episcopalians may abstain from meat on Fridays; communion provided by clergy; anointing of sick may be offered although not required
- *Lutheran* (10 different branches): Communion provided by clergy; anointing of sick by clergy; provide service of Commendation of the Dying
- *Mennonite:* Prayer has important role during crisis or illness, as well as anointing with oil; abstain from alcohol; may oppose medications; women may desire to wear head covering during hospitalization; simple and plain lifestyle and dress style; communion provided twice a year with foot washing part of ceremony
- *Methodist* (more than 20 different groups): Communion provided by clergy; anointing of sick; praying and reading Bible important during illness; organ donation encouraged
- *Presbyterian* (10 different groups): Communion provided by clergy; clergy or elders can provide prayer for the dying
- *Quaker (Friends):* Believe God is personal and real, and that any believer can achieve communion with Jesus Christ without use of clergy or church rituals; no special death ceremony because of belief that present life is part of God's kingdom; abstain from alcohol; may oppose use of medications
- *Seventh-Day Adventist:* Healthy lifestyle practices are promoted, as the body is seen as a temple of the Holy Spirit; alcohol, tobacco, coffee, tea, and recreational drugs are prohibited; pork and shellfish are avoided by most, and many are vegetarians; Sabbath is observed on Saturday; treatment may be opposed on Sabbath; communion provided by clergy; Bible reading important

ROMAN CATHOLICISM: Believe in Jesus Christ as Savior

Believe in Pope as head of the church on Earth; express faith mainly in formulated creeds, such as Apostle's Creed; fasting during Lent and on Fridays optional, although older Catholics may adhere to practice; priest provides communion, Sacrament of the Sick, and hears confession; rosary beads, medals, statues, and other religious objects important

(continued)

TABLE 12.1 Major Religions and Their Practices That May Need to Be Considered in Caregiving (*Continued*)

EASTERN ORTHODOXY: Believe in Jesus Christ as Savior

Includes Greek, Serbian, Russian, and other orthodox churches; believe Holy Spirit proceeds from Father (rather than Father and Son), therefore, reject authority of Pope; fast from meat and dairy products on Wednesdays and Fridays during Lent and on other holy days; follow different calendar for religious celebrations; fast during Lent and before communion; holy unction administered to sick but not necessarily as last rites; last rites must be provided by ordained priest

OTHER CHRISTIAN RELIGIONS

- *Christian Science:* Religion based on use of faith for healing; may decline drugs, psychotherapy, hypnotism, vaccination, and some treatments; use Christian Science nurses and other practitioners and may desire that they be active participants in care
- *Jehovah's Witnesses:* Will not use alcohol and tobacco; blood transfusions not accepted although alternative methods can be used
- *Mormons (Church of Jesus Christ of Latter Day Saints):* No professional clergy; communion and anointing of sick/laying on of hands can be provided by member of church priesthood; abstain from alcohol; discourage use of caffeine, alcohol, and other substances that are considered unhealthy and harmful; a sacred undergarment may be worn at all times that is only removed in absolute emergencies; prayer and reading sacred writings important; may oppose some medical treatments and use divine healing through laying on of hands
- *Unitarian:* Liberal branch of Christianity; belief in God as single being rather than doctrine of the Trinity; believe individuals are responsible for their own health state; advocate donation of body organs

JUDAISM: Believe in one universal God and that Jews were specially chosen to receive God's laws; observe Sabbath from sundown Friday to nightfall Saturday; three branches:

- *Orthodox (observant):* Strictly adhere to traditions of Judaism; believe in divinely inspired five Books of Moses (Torah); follow Kosher diet (no mixing of milk and meat at a meal, no pork or shellfish, no consumption of meat not slaughtered in accordance with Jewish law, use of separate cooking utensils for meat and milk products); strict restrictions during Sabbath (no riding in car, smoking, turning lights on/off, handling money, using telephone or television; medical treatments may be postponed until after Sabbath); men do not shave with razor but may use scissors or electric razor so that blade does not come in contact with skin; men wear skullcaps at all times; beard is considered sign of piety; Orthodox man will not touch any woman other than those in his family; married women cover hair; family and friends visit and may remain with dying person; witness needs to be present when person prays for health so that if death occurs family

TABLE 12.1 Major Religions and Their Practices That May Need to Be Considered in Caregiving *(Continued)*

will be protected by God; after death body should not be left alone and only an Orthodox person should touch or wash body; if death occurs on Sabbath, Orthodox persons cannot handle corpse but nursing staff can care for body wearing gloves; body must be buried within 24 hours; autopsy not allowed; any removed body parts must be returned for burial with the remaining body, as they believe all parts of the body need to be returned to the earth; prayer and quiet time important

- *Conservative:* Follow same basic laws as Orthodox; may only cover heads during worship and prayer; some may approve of autopsy
- *Reformed:* Less stringent adherence to laws; do not strictly follow Kosher diet; do not wear skullcaps; attend temples on Fridays for worship but do not follow restrictions during Sabbath; men can touch women

ISLAM (MUSLIM): Second largest monotheistic (belief in one God) religion; founded by prophet Mohammed who was a human messenger or prophet used by God to communicate His word; Koran is scripture; Koran cannot be touched by anyone ritually unclean and nothing should be placed on Koran; may pray five times a day facing Mecca; privacy during prayer important; abstain from pork and alcohol; all permissible meat must be blessed and killed in special way; cleanliness important; at prayer time, washing is required, even by the sick; accept medical practices if these do not violate religious practices; women are very modest and not allowed to sign consent or make decisions without husband; may wear a *taviz* (black string with words of Koran attached); family or any practicing Muslim can pray with dying person; prefer for family to wash and prepare body of deceased (if necessary, nurses can care for deceased body wearing gloves); autopsy prohibited except when legally mandated; organ donation not allowed

HINDUISM: Considered world's oldest religion; religion of most of India's residents; no scriptures, fixed doctrine, or common worship; belief in karma (every person born into position based on deeds of previous life) and reincarnation; illness may be viewed as result of sin from past life; mostly vegetarian; abstain from alcohol and tobacco

BUDDHISM: Offshoot of Hinduism with most followers in Japan, Thailand, and Myanmar; believe enlightenment found in individual meditation rather than communal worship; follow moral code known as Eightfold Path that leads to nirvana (form of liberation and enlightenment); vegetarian; abstain from alcohol and tobacco; may oppose medications and refuse treatments on holy days; private, uninterrupted time for meditation important

Note: Although the practices are consistent with the religious group, not all individuals who claim to be followers of a specific religion will adhere to all practices.

As the relationship with the patient continues and deepens, spiritual needs that were not revealed during the initial assessment may surface. In addition, the patient may exhibit signs of spiritual distress, which include:

- Crying, sighing
- Anger
- Cynicism, sarcasm
- Depression
- Comments reflecting hopelessness
- Withdrawal
- Apathy, refusal to participate in care
- Sleep disturbances
- Statements questioning one's faith, the presence of God
- Suicidal comments or actions
- Physical symptoms: poor appetite, sleep disturbances, fatigue, sighing

When such signs are present, exploration into the patient's emotional and spiritual state is needed.

ASSISTING WITH SPIRITUAL NEEDS

Plans and actions to address spiritual needs will depend on the cause and the specific spiritual profile of the patient. Interventions that could prove beneficial include:

- *Offering a therapeutic presence:* Being with the patient with the intent to focus on and be available to the patient without performing tasks or being distracted by other activities aids in establishing a therapeutic presence. Conversation can be initiated; however, sometimes sitting in silence may be the best therapeutic action.
- *Respecting beliefs and practices:* Actions such as withholding nonessential activities during times that the patient is praying or engaging in religious activities, assisting the patient in

wearing religious articles, reading to the patient, and honoring the patient's Sabbath facilitate the patient's spiritual health. A patient's personal religious or spiritual belief should not be judged or attempted to be changed by staff.

- *Assisting the patient in meeting religious and spiritual needs:* Assistive actions could include arranging for clergy to visit and helping the patient find transportation to his church or temple.
- *Promoting hope:* Many older adults have challenging lives and health conditions that can shatter optimism and hope. Hope can be promoted by:
  - Developing realistic short-term goals and acknowledging to the patient the achievement of the goals
  - Reinforcing positive outcomes and achievements
  - Engaging in a life review to enable the patient to see the value of his or her life
  - Providing a positive environment (e.g., keeping the room fresh, providing flowers, offering aromatherapy and music)
  - Controlling pain and other symptoms
  - Linking the patient with a support group
  - Suggesting that the patient journal
  - Using humor therapeutically
- *Addressing spiritual distress:* When there is a disruption in the relationship individuals have with spiritual or religious practices, or their spiritual needs are not satisfied, they are in a state of spiritual distress. Factors that contribute to this state include new or worsened illness, losses, inability to engage in religious or spiritual practices, caregiver stress, and feelings that their current problems are the result of sin or inadequate faith. Effective communication skills can assist in assessing factors that contribute to spiritual distress. Once these factors are identified, specific interventions can be planned; these interventions could include referral to clergy/a spiritual leader, assisting with participation in religious or spiritual practices (e.g., reading the Bible, affording periods of solitude), or arranging for prayer. A person's desire *not* to engage in religious practices or to *reject* visits from clergy should be respected, even if this is out of character for the individual.

FAST FACTS in a NUTSHELL

No nurse is expected to engage in a religious activity that violates personal religious beliefs, but if the nurse's and patient's beliefs are similar and the nurse has no objection, the nurse can pray with or for the patient.

As people are spiritual beings, attention to spiritual care is essential. Spiritual well-being can be comforting to patients and provide the strength to enable them to cope with other challenges in their lives.

13

Functional Ability

An important consideration in gerontological nursing care is the older person's ability to perform activities that contribute to independence in daily living and a high quality of life. Aspects of functional independence include bed mobility, transfer, ambulation, hygiene, eating, dressing, dexterity, and use of braces, prostheses, assistive devices, and mobility aids. It also includes a more subtle aspect, being the person's psychological state that affects motivation to achieve the highest potential of functional ability. Nursing must address both physical and psychological factors in promoting maximum functional independence.

All older adults should be encouraged and assisted in functioning at their highest level of ability. This is facilitated by assisting in the identification and reduction of factors that limit independent function. Among these factors could be caregivers' potential for denying the right of these individuals to function at full capacity by performing activities for them that they are able to perform independently if ample time and encouragement are given.

Objectives

In this chapter you will learn to:

1. Describe components of the assessment of functional ability
2. List specific measures to assess activities of daily living and instrumental activities of daily living
3. Describe interventions that could be used to address deficits in functional ability
4. Describe basic range of motion exercises
5. Describe factors to consider in using mobility aids with older adults

ASSESSMENT

FAST FACTS in a NUTSHELL

In restorative and rehabilitative nursing activities, functional capacity yields greater insight into necessary plans and interventions than do diagnoses.

[Clinical Snapshot]

Two older adults visiting the primary care center have similar histories of diabetes mellitus, cardiac disease, and arthritis. One is employed, exercises at a gym a few times weekly, and travels extensively. The other has opted for early retirement and developed a sedentary lifestyle due to viewing himself through his diseases (e.g., I'm a diabetic) and believing he needed to reduce his activity and take extra caution due to his diagnoses. Their similar diagnoses have impacted each of them very differently; therefore, it is essential that the impact of diagnoses on their function be explored when attempting to identify their individual needs and related actions to address them.

Assessment of functional capacity begins at the time of initial contact with the older adult and may require additional assessment thereafter to obtain an accurate view of function. For example, an older person may have difficulty ambulating and dressing himself or herself in the early morning, but as the day progresses and joint function improves he or she may be capable of performing these activities independently. Another individual may appear normal in the ability to function in the morning, but as the day progresses becomes fatigued and helpless. Whenever possible, obtaining a 24-hour profile of function is an ideal way to assess functional ability. This may be possible in a nursing home, hospital, or assisted-living community, but may prove to be more challenging for the older person who lives in the community. For the community-based older person, a history that reviews 24-hour activity and the input of others who live in the same household could provide important information to help assess function effectively.

The range of motion of all joints should be assessed and limitations described as specifically as possible.

Assessment of activities of daily living (ADLs) and instrumental activities of daily living (IADLs) provide the foundation for evaluating functional ability. The following are activities to assess for each of the ADLs:

Mobility
- Bed activities:
  - If the person is lying in bed, ask the patient to roll from side to side, turn from the back to the abdomen, and roll to the back again.
  - Have the person sit up erect in bed and then swing the legs over the side of the bed.
  - Place an object on the night stand and ask the person to reach for it.
- Transfer:
  - Have the person sit on the edge of the bed and then ask the person to stand.
  - Ask the person to sit and then rise from a chair.
  - Observe the person transferring to a commode and tub or shower.

- Ambulation:
  - Have the person walk and observe balance and independence.
  - If a cane is used, observe appropriateness of use and ease of ambulation with its use.
  - Observe the person walking up and down stairs.
  - If a wheelchair is used, note the ability to propel the wheelchair and apply its brakes.

Bathing
- Observe strength of upper extremities.
- Note ability to lift arm to face and head.
- Note ability to manage a razor and comb hair.
- Observe ability to handle soap and washcloth.
- Observe ability to turn faucets.

Dressing
- Determine ability to put on and remove all clothing.
- Observe dexterity with zippers, buttons, snaps, and shoelaces.

Eating
- Observe ability to grip and use each utensil.
- Note ability to cut foods, open containers, and hold a cup/glass.

Toileting
- Observe ability to use a commode or bedpan.
- Note the ability to use toilet tissue to perform hygienic techniques.

FAST FACTS in a NUTSHELL

The Katz Index of Independence in Daily Living has been an accepted tool for assessing ADLs for decades. This easy-to-use tool scores each of the ADLs to determine a person's degree of dependence or independence. A sample of the tool can be viewed at the Harford Institute for Geriatric Nursing. Try this webpage: consultgerirn.org/uploads/File/trythis/try_this_2.pdf.

The performance of IADLs is more significant to the older adult who is residing in the community; this also is significant if the person in a nursing home or assistive living community is planning to be discharged to the community. In assessing IADLs, determine the following:

- *Ability to use a telephone:* Note ability to dial numbers and answer the phone.
- *Shopping:* Determine degree of independence in shopping for needs.
- *Food preparation:* Note the ability to plan, prepare, and serve meals.
- *Housekeeping:* Determine ability to maintain home and perform basic tasks, such as dishwashing and bed making.
- *Laundry:* Review degree to which personal laundry can be done independently.
- *Transportation:* Note ability to travel independently on public transportation or drive a car.
- *Medications:* Determine the degree to which the person can be responsible for taking medication in correct dose at correct times.
- *Money management:* Review ability to manage financial matters, such as writing checks, paying bills, tracking income and expenses, and banking.

FAST FACTS in a NUTSHELL

There are several tools available to assist in assessing IADLs. The Instrumental Activities of Daily Living Scale (Lawton and Brody, 1969) has long been used to score IADL independence. The Cleveland Scale for Activities of Daily Living (CSADL) is an informant-based instrument that expands existing ADL and IADL instruments and is particularly useful in assessing ADL and IADL capacity in persons with dementia (Patterson & Mack, 2001).

DECONDITIONING AND SARCOPENIA

Deconditioning refers to the multiple changes in the body systems that occur as a result of inactivity. Impaired physical mobility, immobility, and disuse syndrome are terms that are sometimes used to describe deconditioning. Deconditioning can take the form of:

- *Acute deconditioning:* This happens rapidly as a result of a sudden cessation of usual activity. This can occur when a person fractures a hip, is hospitalized, and inactive for a period of time.
- *Chronic deconditioning:* This is a slower process in which there is a gradual reduction in activity over time. This can develop when a person reduces ambulation due to increased arthritis pain or when grief causes a person to withdraw and reduce activity.

As psychosocial factors can contribute to deconditioning, the importance of identifying all factors that could impact health status cannot be overstated.

Sarcopenia, a decrease in muscle mass and/or function resulting from a reduction of protein synthesis and an increase in muscle protein degradation, can contribute to impaired function. Immobility and lack of exercise, increased levels of proinflammatory cytokines, increased production of oxygen free radicals or impaired detoxification, low anabolic hormone output, malnutrition, and reduced neurological drive have been advocated as being responsible for sarcopenia (Di Iorio et al., 2006). When added to the impaired capacity for muscle regeneration that occurs in late life, this can lead to disability, particularly when compounded by diseases or organ impairment. The deconditioning effects of inactivity are significant in older adults and exaggerate the effects of sarcopenia, so every effort must be made to maximize their activity level.

INTERVENTIONS

The primary goal in assisting older adults with functional ability is to maximize independence. Efforts to preserve and use existing function are an important aspect of this. Patients should be encouraged to be as independent as possible and receive positive reinforcement offered when they are. Simple acts by patients, such as combing one's hair or performing a partial bath, should be recognized; although seemingly simple, they could have required considerable effort to complete. Caregivers need to understand that although more time may be needed, patients need to be given the opportunity to engage in ADLs and IADLs as independently as possible.

When deficits in performing activities are present, consider the type of intervention that may be necessary, which could include:

- Education as to alternative ways to perform the activity or measures to reduce the limitation
- Referral for therapy
- Techniques to motivate the person to function to capacity
- Mechanical assistance (e.g., special eating utensils, modified clothing, cane, wheelchair, bedside commode)
- Partial assistance
- Total assistance

Physical and occupational therapists can provide therapies and devices that can enhance independent function significantly. Their inclusion in the plan and support of their recommendations are beneficial.

Range-of-Motion Exercises

Range-of-motion exercises promote joint motion, strengthen muscles, enhance circulation, and assist in the prevention of complications. These exercises can be done:

- Independently, in which the person performs the exercises with no assistance
- With partial assistance (e.g., supporting a limb or helping with a position change)
- With total assistance, whereby the there is no active effort by the individual as the nurse exercises the joint

Basic exercises consist of:

- *Flexion:* bending at the joint
- *Extension:* straightening
- *Abduction:* moving a limb outward, away from the body
- *Adduction:* moving a limb inward, toward the body
- *Internal rotation:* turning the limb inward, toward center
- *External rotation:* turning the limb outward, from center
- *Eversion:* turning the joint outward
- *Circumduction:* moving in a circular manner
- *Pronation:* rotating down, toward back of body
- *Supination:* rotating up, toward front of body

When assisting with range-of-motion exercises, it is important to:

- Support below and above the joint
- Move the joint slowly
- During each exercise session, exercise the joint at least 3 times
- Not force the joint past the point of resistance
- Note any pain, resistance, or abnormal movement (see Table 13.1)
- Document the degree of joint mobility

TABLE 13.1 Signs to Note During Exercise

The following signs could indicate that exercise is not being well tolerated. If any of the signs are present, stop the exercise, evaluate the person, and allow the person to rest.

- Dyspnea
- Pallor, cyanosis
- Dizziness, poor coordination
- Diaphoresis
- Acute confusion, restlessness
- Heart rate during exercise greater than or equal to 35% above the resting heart rate
- Resting heart rate greater than or equal to 100 bpm
- Increase or decrease in systolic blood pressure by 20 mmHg
- Angina

FAST FACTS in a NUTSHELL

In addition to exercise, proper positioning has a role in improving function. When the body is in correct alignment the body systems can function more effectively and contractures and other complications can be avoided. Consideration should be given to proper positioning in chairs and wheelchairs, in addition to the bed.

Mobility Aids

Canes, walkers, and wheelchairs can enhance independence in older adults who have mobility limitations. They also can present safety risks and reduce function if used improperly; therefore, nurses need to ensure the proper use of these aids. Some considerations include:

- Ensure the right type and size of aid is used. Physical therapists can assist with proper measurement and identification of the best aid based on the individual's function. They can also instruct the individual in the proper use of the aid.
- Canes offer the user a wider based of support. They are individually fitted, usually based on the distance from the greater trochanter to a point 6 inches from the side of the person's foot. They are held on the unaffected side and advanced when the affected leg advances. Canes should not be used for bearing weight.
- Walkers provide a base of support and stability due to their ability to bear weight. They are sized by measuring the distance of the trochanter to the floor; the person's elbows should be slightly flexed when standing and holding the sides of the walker. To use the walker the person advances it and then steps forward. When lowering to a chair, the person should step backward until he or she touches the seat, grab the arms of the chair, and lower him- or herself. When rising from a chair, the person should push on the arms of the chair and not attempt to use the walker to lift up.
- Wheelchairs should be individually fitted so that the seat is slightly wider than the person's body and the arms can easily reach the wheels.

Other Aids

There are a variety of aids that can increase independence, such as:

- Easy-grip utensils
- Bedside commodes
- Adjustable height toilet seats
- Lift chairs
- Clothing with Velcro fasteners
- Telephone amplifiers and dial enlargers
- Tub grab bars
- Emergency alarm systems

Occupational and physical therapists are excellent resources for aids that can enhance an older adult's function and independence. For the older person living in the community, home health nurses can assist in helping the person modify the home to promote safe, independent function and to obtain equipment and aids.

OTHER CONSIDERATIONS

Physical condition is a major factor affecting an individual's ability to function, but other factors also play a role. In addition to physical ability, people need to have the following to engage in activities:

- Motivation and desire
- Mental capacity
- Knowledge and skill

People who are depressed may lack the emotional energy to learn to use new devices or participate in therapies. Some individuals may be reluctant to improve function after rehabilitation due to fear of re-injuring themselves or aggravating their condition; overprotective family members may discourage efforts toward patients' more independent function out of similar fears.

━━━━━━━━━━━━━━━ *FAST FACTS in a NUTSHELL*

In some circumstances, people may find it more advantageous to not improve independence.

[Clinical Snapshot]

Seventy-eight-year-old Mrs. H is staying with her daughter's family following a stroke. She enjoys this arrangement, finding her new living conditions superior to when she had been living alone. The home health nurse and physical therapist have been concerned that Mrs. H has not made the expected recovery of function. In exploring reasons for her lack of progress, a factor to consider is that although she has the physical capacity to function more independently, she lacks the desire to do so and intentionally has resisted following through on recommended exercises that could increase her function. It could be that Mrs. H perceives that it is not in her best interest to engage in rehabilitation to increase her independence, as this would cause her to be able to return to her home. These types of factors need to be evaluated when progress seems unusually delayed or in developing discharge plans.

To understand the benefits of efforts to improve functional ability, follow instructions for exercises, use assistive devices and mobility aids correctly, and otherwise comply with restorative and rehabilitative measures people need the ability to understand, interpret, and follow directions. This relies on good cognitive function. Individuals with dementia, for example, may not have the capacity to remember how to use a walker properly or when to do their exercises, and they may resist rehabilitative efforts because they lack the mental capacity to appreciate the benefits.

For many people, improving or restoring function requires that they learn new knowledge and skills. Seemingly simple acts, such as walking with a cane or transferring from the bed to a chair involve specific steps in order to be done correctly. Gaining the new knowledge and skills are important to the ability of older adults to improve function. Patient teaching is an important component of rehabilitative efforts; nurses need to:

- *Assess learning needs:* There can be variation in the knowledge and skills individuals require. For example, one patient may be familiar with exercises or assistive devices because she helped her husband with them after his stroke several years previously. One patient may be totally unfamiliar with measures needed to improve function while another may have done extensive research and have a good understanding.
- *Develop individualized teaching plans:* In addition to the content that needs to be addressed, consideration must be given to the level of instruction that is appropriate for the individual, readiness to learn, factors that could interfere with learning, and language barriers. Ask the patient if there is any other person that he or she would want to have present during the instruction or to whom instruction should be provided.
- *Supplement verbal instruction:* For anyone, there is a risk that verbal instructions may not be properly heard or may be forgotten; when a person is of advanced age, has multiple health conditions, or may be experiencing side effects of medications, the risk of verbal instruction not being understood or remembered is high. It is useful to offer written instructions and fact sheets to supplement verbal instruction.
- *Move at the individual's pace:* Fatigue, pain, short attention spans, feelings of being overwhelmed, and other factors can cause people to become overwhelmed and block out information. Pay attention to the patient's response and adjust instruction to accommodate the patient's readiness and tolerance.
- *Evaluate the patient's understanding:* Ask for feedback and return demonstrations to ensure the patient has grasped the instruction. Encourage the patient to ask to have instruction repeated if needed.
- *Document:* Be sure to note in the record the information taught and the patient's response.

There are many factors that can threaten functional ability in late life. It is important for the gerontological nurse to consider these factors and assess the level of independence of older patients. When independent function of older patients is threatened, nurses need to ensure actions are taken to improve functional ability. As the status of older adults can change over time, reassessment and revision of goals and plans may be necessary.

14

Safety

Safety is a concern for persons of all ages; however, in late life a variety of factors heighten safety risks. The injury rate for persons age 65 and older falls in the midrange for people of all age groups until age 75 and older, when it rises, thereby causing persons over age 75 to have the second highest rate of injury. Injuries rank in the top ten leading causes of death for persons over age 65 (Chen, Warner, Fingerhut, & Makur, 2009).

A major factor affecting safety of older adults is the impact of aging changes, such as:

- *Poorer vision: labels may be misread, changes in walking surfaces unnoticed, hazards not seen, and vision diminished in poorly lit areas and at night*
- *Poorer hearing: smoke detectors, alarms, and other warnings may be missed*
- *Altered center of gravity: balance is lost more easily*
- *Delayed response and reaction time: slower ability to regain balance after losing it, which increases risk for falling*
- *Demineralization of bone: fractures occur more easily*
- *Poorer memory: instructions may not be remembered, items cooking on the stove may be forgotten*

In addition to age-related changes, the high prevalence of chronic diseases can contribute to safety risks. The medications

> used to treat these conditions can cause dizziness, drowsiness, orthostatic hypotension, incontinence, and other side effects that can cause falls and other injuries. There is a high prevalence of the use of canes, walkers, and wheelchairs; if used improperly these aids can contribute to falls. The high rate of altered cognition in the older population heightens safety risks. The significant risks that are present in the older population demand that nurses be attentive to preventing injuries and complications.

Objectives

In this chapter you will learn to:

1. Describe factors leading to increased safety risks in older adults
2. Describe environmental risks to the safety of older adults
3. List interventions that could assist in reducing falls
4. Describe factors to consider in assessing for potential risks related to medications
5. Describe reasons for infections being more challenging for older adults
6. Identify factors that heighten the risk for older drivers to have accidents

ENVIRONMENTAL CONSIDERATIONS

Age-related changes and the effects of diseases may pose safety risks that nurses are limited in eliminating; however, there are actions nurses can take to reduce risks that are external to the individual. Sensitivity to aspects of the environment that impact safety and reducing environmental risks are essential components of geriatric care.Specific considerations include:

- *Lighting.* Older eyes are particularly sensitive to glare. Common sources of glare are fluorescent lights, sunlight, and highly polished or high-gloss surfaces of floors and furniture. Glare from these sources can be reduced by:

- Using several diffuse sources of lighting rather than single bright lights
- Filtering incoming sunlight from windows with the use of sheer curtains or adjusted blinds
- Avoiding floor polishing
- Selecting furniture that does not have high-gloss finishes
- It takes longer for older eyes to adjust from dark to light areas, so abrupt changes in lighting should be avoided. The use of nightlights can avoid dramatic changes in lighting and provide light for older adults who need to use the bathroom during the night.

- *Color.* The yellowing of the lens that occurs with age can affect the perception of blue and green colors. Older eyes can have difficulty differentiating among various shades of blues and greens. For example, if the flooring is green and the upholstery on the chair is another shade of green, the older person may misjudge the edge of the chair and slip to the floor. Likewise, if the floor has blue carpeting and the stairway has another shade of blue carpeting, the older individual may not notice the change in level and fall down the steps. Blue print on green paper can be difficult for the older adult to read, causing instructions to be missed. If blues and greens are used, there should be good color contrast with the use of other colors.

- *Floor coverings.* Carpeting presents many problems in environments in which older adults live, such as:
  - Static cling
  - Difficulty cleaning and eliminating odors
  - Difficulty with wheelchair mobility
  - Haven for cockroaches, moths, and other pests on the undersurface
  - Scattered and area rugs can be a source of falls, as well. Non-glare tiled floors, ideally with nonslip surface finishes, are best for the environments of older persons.

  - *Bathroom.* Bathrooms can be extremely hazardous places for older persons. Wet floors can contribute to slips and falls, and the hard surfaces that can be struck during a fall can heighten the risk of serious injury. Care must be taken to avoid leaving towels, hairdryers, and other items on the floor.

- Tubs and showers should have nonslip surfaces. Shower and bath seats can offer a means to rest if fatigue or dizziness occurs. Grab bars and safety rails can be useful in providing added stability.
- The slower reaction times of older adults can prevent them from withdrawing quickly from water that is excessively hot. Having centrally controlled hot water temperatures can aid in reduce the risk of burns.
- It is beneficial to avoid using electric heaters, radios, hair dryers, and other electrical appliances in the bathroom. Even a person in good physical condition could accidentally slip and sustain a burn or electrical shock.

- *Fires.* Older persons living in the community who independently cook should be advised to set the timer when using the oven or stovetop as a means to not forget that they have something cooking. Persons with gas burners need to be cautioned about the risk of bathrobe sleeves and loose clothing catching on fire as they reach across the stovetop.
- The environment should be inspected for overloaded electrical receptacles. In some cases, this occurs because the older person cannot reach behind furniture to use other outlets; assisting in finding additional outlets to use may be needed.
- Smoking carries many risks; one of which is the potential of a carelessly disposed of lit match or cigarette butt causing a fire. Older smokers should be advised to smoke in a safe place, such as a patio, and cautioned about safety.

FAST FACTS in a NUTSHELL

In health care facilities, additional safety risks can present, such as unlocked medication carts, cleaning solutions, walk-in freezers, and pushes and shoves from other patients. The impact of these risks on individual patients should be considered and specific plans developed to address them.

- *Clutter.* Years of accumulating and limited energy or ability to sort, store, and dispose of items can cause the homes of some older adults to be quite cluttered. This poses problems in terms of cleanliness, fire hazards, and falls. If older adults are unable to organize and clean their homes, family members or church or other volunteer groups should be recruited to assist.

FALLS

Of all injuries, fall-related injuries are the major cause of hospitalization, traumatic brain injuries, and fractures. Over the past decade, the death rate from falls has risen sharply (Centers for Disease Control and Prevention [CDC], 2011). Even if physical injury does not result from a fall, many older adults who have had a fall will limit their activities due to concerns of falling again; this unnecessarily can reduce their activity, socialization, and quality of life. These realities emphasize the need for nurses to be proactive in helping older adults prevent falls and effectively managing them when they do occur.

FAST FACTS in a NUTSHELL

Approximately one third of people over the age of 65 experience a fall each year, and as many as 30% of those who fall suffer moderate to severe injuries that can threaten their independence and quality of life (CDC, 2012).

Fall risk should be incorporated into the assessment of older adults. Some of the factors that can heighten the risk for falling are listed in Table 14.1. Specifically identifying risks can guide the development of effective plans and actions, which could include measures such as:

- Referring to physical therapy for instruction on transfer techniques or proper use of mobility aids
- Strengthening exercises

TABLE 14.1 Factors Increasing the Risk for Falls

- Being a woman 75 years of age or older
- A history of falls
- Use of cane, walker, wheelchair, brace
- Presence of a physical disability
- Multiple diagnoses
- Cerebrovascular accident, transient ischemic attack
- Unstable cardiac condition
- Neurological disease
- Musculoskeletal condition, foot problems
- Presence of a dementia, delirium, or mood disturbance
- Hypotension
- Dizziness, weakness, fatigue
- Paralysis
- Edema
- New environment
- Use of antidepressants, antihypertensives, antipsychotics, diuretics, sedatives, tranquilizers, multiple medications
- Environmental risks: scatter rugs, highly polished floors, poor lighting, absence of railings and grab bars, pets

- Medication change
- Reinforcement of need to change positions slowly
- Improved management of medical condition
- Provision of assistance with transfers and ambulation
- Referral for eye examination and/or new eyeglass prescription
- Altering home environment to remove obstacles from walking path

Be it the person's home in the community or a health care facility, the environment used by the older adult should be evaluated for factors that can contribute to falls. This could include clutter on the floor, glare created from unfiltered sunlight coming through a window, poorly lit stairways, or leaks causing slippery surfaces. Caregivers need to be advised of environmental factors contributing to falls and guided in reducing them.

When a fall occurs, the person should be kept immobile until a full examination for injury is performed. Items to note include:

- Skin breaks
- Discoloration

- Bleeding
- Swelling
- Asymmetry of extremities
- Abnormal appearance or loss of function of affected area
- Pain

================================== *FAST FACTS in a NUTSHELL*

In some older adults, a fracture may not be readily apparent following a fall. Later, when the person resumes normal activity, signs may be noted. This emphasizes the need to observe the person carefully over the next 24 hours following a fall to detect injuries.

Examination needs to be done not just of the body part that struck the surface during the fall, but all potential sites of impact. For example, a person may have fallen on the knee, but the impact could have placed sufficient pressure on the hip to cause a fracture at that site as well. If there is any suspicion of injury, the person should be evaluated.

Interventions related to the specific factors that contributed to the fall should be planned to avoid future falls; these could include:

- Orienting patients to new environments, including location of emergency call signals, exits, light switches, and stairwells
- Ensuring patients are wearing prescribed eyeglasses and hearing aids
- Ensuring canes, walkers, and wheelchairs are readily accessible and properly used
- Observing patients' clothing and shoes for potential risks (e.g., pant legs dragging floor, loose slippers)
- Keeping walking areas clutter-free and dry
- Providing ample lighting; preventing glare
- Encouraging patients to use grab bars and hand rails
- Keeping medications and noningestible solutions properly stored

- Cleaning spills promptly
- Promptly reporting plumbing leaks, broken equipment, and other maintenance problems
- Observing for changes in status and function that could heighten the risk for falls (e.g., blood pressure changes, dizziness, incontinence, delirium)

MEDICATIONS

The older population uses a large number and variety of medications that increase their risk for adverse drug reactions and administration errors.

FAST FACTS in a NUTSHELL

The most commonly used medications among older adults are cardiovascular agents, antihypertensives, analgesics, antiarthritic agents, sedatives, tranquilizers, laxatives, and antacids. Many of these drugs can produce confusion, dizziness, and weakness as adverse effects, which can threaten safety.

During the assessment, all medications used by the older person should be reviewed with attention to:

- *The reason the medication is being used.* A person may have been prescribed a sedative months ago after the death of a spouse, but now that she is adjusting to widowhood may not require the sleep aid.
- *The appropriateness of the dosage.* As the person has aged or lost weight, the dose that was prescribed several years ago may be too high and require adjustment.
- *The manner in which the medication is being administered.* Ensure that enteric-coated tablets are not being crushed, drugs that should be taken with meals are not taken first thing in the morning on an empty stomach, and that medications that should not be administered concurrently are being taken together.

- *The effects of the medication.* It is not only important to determine if medications are producing adverse effects, but also if they are having the intended effect.

When reviewing the medications used by older adults it is important to remember potentially inappropriate drugs that should be avoided in this population (see Chapter 16).

Identifying and correcting medication-related problems discovered during the assessment can prevent complications that can threaten safety and well-being.

To promote medication self-administration safety, a detailed description, both verbal and written, should be given to patients and their caregivers, outlining the:

- Drug's name
- Dosage
- Route of administration
- Action
- Special precautions
- Incompatible foods or drugs
- Adverse reactions

FAST FACTS in a NUTSHELL

Some of the common self-medication errors that occur with older adults include incorrect dosage, noncompliance arising from misunderstanding, discontinuation or unnecessary continuation of drugs without medical advice, and the use of medications prescribed for previous illnesses. Anticipating these and providing education to reduce the risks of them occurring are necessary.

A color-coded dosage schedule can be developed to assist persons who have limited vision or who are unable to read instructions. Medication labels with large print and caps that can be easily removed by weak or arthritic hands should be provided.

Additional information on medication safety can be found in Chapter 16.

INFECTIONS

Infections are a significant risk for older adults due to age-related changes that cause the body to be more prone to develop infections and the high prevalence of chronic conditions. Consider that:

- Pneumonia is a leading cause of infection-related death; older individuals have a threefold greater incidence of nosocomial pneumonia as compared to younger age groups.
- Older adults experience gastroenteritis caused by *Salmonella* species more frequently than persons younger than 65 years of age.
- More than half of all reported cases of tetanus, endocarditis, cholelithiasis, and diverticulitis occur among older persons.

Not only do infections occur more frequently among older adults, but they are often delayed in being detected due to altered symptomatology. For example, lower normal body temperatures in older persons can cause fever to appear at levels that may not be considered significant for younger persons, and, consequently, not addressed. Likewise, altered pain sensations can cause pneumonia or appendicitis to be present without the signs of pain common in younger populations. Special attention is needed to reduce the older person's contact with persons who have infections, and help the older person enhance immunity and maintain a healthy body to be able to resist infections.

OLDER DRIVERS

FAST FACTS in a NUTSHELL

As a group, persons over age 60 have a lower rate of driving accidents; however:
- Car accident rates increase after age 75
- Persons age 85 and older have four times the number of accidents on a mile-per-driven basis as compared to persons aged 50 to 59
- Older adults are 15 times more likely to die in car accidents as compared to drivers in their 40s (Shallenbarger, 2012).

There are rising numbers of older drivers on the road who can potentially pose a safety risk to themselves and others. Consider that older drivers often have:

- Poorer vision
- Slower response and reaction times
- Side effects from medications that can affect mental clarity and physical function
- Health conditions that can create symptoms when these individuals are behind the wheel

Although driving safety can vary among individuals, older adults should be aided in evaluating their competencies behind the wheel. Specific questions that can aid in this review include:

- Are you able to apply the brakes quickly?
- Do you have difficulty driving in bright sunlight or at night?
- Can you adequately see traffic in other lanes when trying to change lanes?
- Do you have difficulty judging parking spaces?
- Can you adequately see what is behind you when pulling out of parking spaces in parking lots?
- Do you find that you have trouble concentrating on your driving or handling the car when you are feeling stressed?
- Do you have any trouble pumping gas into your car?
- Do you find that you get a little disoriented or lost when driving to familiar places?

Responses to these questions can aid in identifying specific safety risks that need to be addressed. Local chapters of the Automobile Association of America (AAA), AARP, and senior citizen groups often sponsor safe driving classes that could prove useful for older drivers.

15

Family Health

A common feature of all human beings is that they are a product of some type of family unit. From the family, individuals gain identity and status, and learn values, beliefs, and attitudes. The family can nurture or harm, promote wellness or pathology, and provide strong support or chronic distress.

The assumption is sometimes made that the presence of family members means that the older adult has support and assistance. However, the existence of family members does not necessarily mean there is a healthy or close relationship, or that there is an ability of family members to have a role in the older adult's life. Nor does it mean that the older individual desires to receive aid from, share problems with, or live with family members. In some circumstances, family members can be a burden and source of problems for the older adults, rather than a joy and source of support. It is essential to assess family dynamics and health when caring for the older person.

Objectives

In this chapter you will learn to:

1. Identify the variety of family structures in which older adults can live
2. Describe the realities of caregiving responsibilities in the United States
3. List components of a family assessment
4. List the types of interventions that can be used to address the family's problems and needs
5. Identify signs of elder abuse and neglect

ROLES, RELATIONSHIPS, AND RESPONSIBILITIES

The meaning of family can vary with the major transformations that family structures have experienced. In the last half century alone, this diversity has grown significantly. The once common nuclear family consisting of a man, woman, and their children has given away to family structures of single parents, same-sex couples, same-sex couples with children, blended families, couples without children, and grandparents raising grandchildren. Today's family structure is also impacted by couples dissolving their relationships and entering new ones more frequently than previous generations. These diverse family structures can impact the availability of caregivers for older adults, as well as their responsibilities to their families.

The practice of women marrying men older than themselves and outliving their spouses results in more older women living alone than older men. This does not mean women are without family support. Most older people have regular contact with family members, and families do provide a variety of assistance to older members, ranging from financial assistance to transportation to health provider visits to personal care (see Box 15.1). In turn, older adults provide assistance and support to their younger family members, such as shared housing, financial assistance, and raising grandchildren. These realities reinforce the necessity of considering the family when assessing, planning, and delivering care.

FAST FACTS in a NUTSHELL

For older adults living in the community, most care is provided by family members, not formal agencies. The realities are:

- *An estimated 10 million people provide care for their parents and approximately half of these engage in parent care on a regular basis.*
- *Wives constitute half of the caregivers for older adults, with daughters and daughters-in-law representing the next largest group.*
- *Women today who provide parent care will spend more time doing so than they spent caring for their own children. Many of these women may still be raising their own children while providing parent care and in some cases raising grandchildren.*
- *A considerable number of caregivers are employed full time in addition to family responsibilities.*
- *Nearly half of the caregivers of older adults are over the age of 65 years themselves.*

Box 15.1   Examples of Assistance That Family Members Can Offer to Older Relatives

- Accompaniment to appointments (e.g., health care provider, financial officers, attorneys)
- Caregiving (e.g., administering medications and treatments, bathing, dressing, feeding)
- Crisis management (e.g., supporting through hospitalization, assisting with relocation, settling family conflict)
- Decision-making assistance
- Education (e.g., medications, use of new appliances/technology, health care practices)
- Emotional support
- Financial management (e.g., managing bank accounts, paying bills, investing)
- Home maintenance

(continued)

Box 15.1   (Continued)

- Housekeeping
- Meal preparation or provision
- Monitoring medications
- Planning and organizing affairs (legal documents, funeral arrangements)
- Respite from caregiving responsibilities
- Shopping
- Socialization
- Telephone contact (e.g., daily checks, reminders to take medications)
- Transportation

It is often assumed that because an older adult has a spouse or children, the family will provide necessary caregiving functions. However, the availability of family members does not mean that the family can be depended upon for assistance and caregiving. There are a variety of reasons why a family may not assist an older relative, including the family member's own poor health, personal burdens, work responsibilities, lack of skill, discomfort with caregiving, poor relationship with the older relative, history of mistreatment by the older relative, and opposition from the family member's spouse. These factors need to be explored during the assessment.

FAST FACTS in a NUTSHELL

Support and caregiving assistance can come from sources other than immediate relatives. Friends, neighbors, church members, and distant relatives may play an important role in the older person's life.

FAMILY ASSESSMENT

Assessing the family structure and dynamics not only helps in identifying potential sources of support and assistance, but also in recognizing potential sources of burdens and problems for the older individual. For example, an older man may have unexplained weight loss. In discussing his family situation it may be discovered that he is so exhausted from caring for his disabled wife that he doesn't take time to properly eat. Rather than diagnostic testing, he may be better served by having caregiver assistance and home-delivered meals provided. Likewise, it may be discovered that an older woman's refusal to agree to surgery is due to the fact that she is the primary caregiver for three young grandchildren whose parents have abandoned them. Assisting her in finding responsible caregivers for her grandchildren while she has surgery could yield a better outcome than continued explanations of the importance of the surgery.

Factors to consider when performing a family assessment with an older adult are:

- Family members with whom the older person has regular contact, a relationship, and frequency of contact
- Persons living in the same household
- If married, health of and relationship with spouse
- The older adult's role and responsibilities in the family
- Quality of family relationships
- Type of assistance provided by family members (see Box 15.1)
- Family members whom the older person would like to have informed and involved in care
- Person who helps the older person make decisions
- Family members dependent on the older person and nature of dependency
- Family members of whom the older adult is afraid or was mistreated by
- Conflict within the family that affects the older person
- Concerns or problems related to family members
- Significant others who provide support and assistance
- Involvement with faith communities, local organizations

The information obtained through this assessment can be valuable in identifying potential problems that may need to be addressed, such as suspected abuse or the need for financial aid for the family unit, as well as issues that may need to be addressed to enable the family to assist in caregiving functions.

FAST FACTS in a NUTSHELL

The importance of the older adult within the family can be highlighted to motivate that individual to comply with health plans and engage in self-care.

INTERVENTIONS

A variety of interventions can be employed to address problems and needs identified through the assessment, such as:

- *Provision of information:* Family members engaged in the care of the older adult can benefit from a review of the diagnoses of the older adult, treatments, precautions, prognosis, and available resources. To abide by laws related to privacy and confidentiality of health care information, the older adult, if not competent to grant consent of his or her legal representative, should be asked if such a discussion with family members is desired and, if so, grant written consent for this information to be shared. (Check your organization's policy regarding this.)
- *Family meetings:* With the older adult's or legal representative's consent, conduct a meeting in which care needs, goals, and plans are discussed. During this meeting family members can share their abilities or limitations to assist.
- *Resident and family education:* The older person and his or her caregivers can be taught the specific skills and knowledge required to provide necessary care. Printed literature and written instructions should be provided for future reference.
- *Referral to resources:* Information about community resources that can provide assistance, the scope of their services, and costs should be reviewed. The nurse can initiate the referral

FAST FACTS in a NUTSHELL

The nurse may be able to address topics during family meetings that the older person and other family members may be reluctant to introduce.

[**Clinical Snapshot**]

Ms. G is a single woman who lives within several miles of her widowed 84-year-old mother. She has three sisters and a brother, who are all married and live anywhere from one half to 1 hour away. Although she has a demanding career and active social life, Ms. G attempts to help her mother; however, lately, the demands of assisting her mother with personal care and maintaining her home have increased to the point that daily assistance is needed. Ms. G has mentioned this to her siblings who have expressed appreciation for what Ms. G is doing, but fail to offer help.

Recognizing this situation, the visiting nurse helps Ms. G to see how it is in her and her mother's best interest to obtain assistance from her siblings. If after offering specific suggestions on the type of help that can be requested the nurse finds that Ms. G still feels uncomfortable addressing the topic, a family meeting could be planned in which the nurse introduces and guides this discussion of greater shared responsibilities for the mother's care.

if the family agrees. The availability of support groups in the community should be provided, including their meeting times and locations.

The nurse should monitor the older adult and his or her family to evaluate the ongoing effectiveness of plans and to identify problems, such as:

- *Poor quality of care*: The older recipient of care may show indications that hygienic needs are not being met, weight loss is occurring, medications are not being properly administered, and complications are developing. Poor quality of care can be the result of the needs of the resident increasing, the caregiving demands being excessive for the caregiver, declining health of the caregiver, or conflict between the caregiver and the older person.
- *Declining health or quality of life of the caregiver*: The resident may be receiving proper care and thriving at the expense of the caregiver's health.

- *Added family burdens:* A caregiver daughter may have recently acquired the responsibility of caring for grandchildren, thereby threatening her ongoing ability to fulfill caregiver functions for the older adult.
- *Changing financial status:* Family members may have been able to manage caregiving responsibilities effectively with the help of a home health aide who provided assistance on mornings while they were at work; however, the older adult and family members may no longer be able to afford this service, leaving a gap in caregiving services.
- *Abuse and neglect:* Caregiver stress, poor quality of relationships, and emotional problems of family members can contribute to abuse. Abuse can take many forms (see Box 15.2) and may not be readily apparent due to the older adult's reluctance to admit mistreatment or the attributing of injuries and other problems to the health status of the older person. Protecting the older adult is the top priority. Nurses should appreciate that in some circumstances abusive behaviors may have been present in the family for a long time and hidden by the older adult. Older adults may not admit abuse or deny it is present due to embarrassment, fear that this could anger their abusers and cause greater problems, or concern that the alternative (e.g., relocation to a nursing home) would be a less desirable situation.

Box 15.2   Elder Mistreatment

Mistreatment of older adults can take the form of:

- *Physical abuse:* infliction of physical pain or injury (e.g., kicking, punching, burning, restraining)
- *Emotional abuse:* infliction of fear, distress, anxiety, or psychological anguish (e.g., threatening, intimidating, verbal abuse)
- *Financial abuse:* misusing the older person's money or property (e.g., stealing money, theft, forgery of documents, transferring or withdrawing investments without consent)

(continued)

- *Sexual abuse*: having sexual contact without consent (e.g., rape, photographing the person nude, forcing the person to perform sexual acts, unwanted touching of genitalia)
- *Neglect*: abandoning or failing to provide necessary food, fluid, hygienic care, medications, treatments, and protection to a person for whom one is responsible

Signs of mistreatment can include:

- Unexplained bruises, cuts, fractures
- Vaginal bleeding or tears
- Change in behavior or mood (e.g., anxiety, withdrawal, agitation, depression)
- Sudden change in financial status, concerns over unpaid bills
- Malnutrition
- Lack of cleanliness in dependent person
- Unclean or unsafe home, roach or rodent infestation
- Overmedication, nonadherence to medication or treatment schedule
- Reluctance to openly talk in the presence of family member or caregiver

Questions that can assist in revealing possible mistreatment include:

- Has anyone harmed you or threatened to harm you?
- Is there anyone whom you are afraid of?
- Are you being adequately cared for?
- Did anyone touch you inappropriately or attempt to have sex with you against your wishes?
- Has anyone made comments to you that caused you to be uncomfortable or afraid?
- Do you have any concern about how your caregiver or relative is handling your money?
- Have you discovered any of your possessions or money missing?
- Have you been forced to do anything that you didn't want to do or that made you uncomfortable?

(continued)

Box 15.2   (Continued)

It is useful to interview the older person alone as the family member accompanying the person may be the perpetrator of the mistreatment and this could discourage the older person from giving honest responses.

Responses that suggest possible or actual abuse should be further explored as to the nature of the mistreatment and the perpetrator. The most common perpetrators are:

- Family members
- Caregivers
- Persons with a history of strained relationships with the older person
- Persons with emotional/psychiatric problems

Interventions when mistreatment is suspected or confirmed include:

- Establish trust with the older adult
- Provide the person with information on reporting the mistreatment or if the person is unable to do so independently, report the mistreatment to appropriate state agency. The National Center for Elder Abuse of the Administration on Aging offers guidance on finding the appropriate reporting agency and other resources within each state on their website: www.ncea.aoa.gov.
- Engage the interdisciplinary team to develop a comprehensive plan for addressing the results of the mistreatment and preventing it in the future.

FAST FACTS in a NUTSHELL

Persons with dementia are a high-risk group for elder mistreatment by their caregivers due to the stress and demands they place on their caregivers. As they may have difficulty reporting mistreatment, special attention is needed to identify indications of this problem. In addition, interventions, such as respite care, should be planned to prevent caregiver burnout that could lead to mistreatment.

As an older adult's condition declines, or changes in mood or cognition occur, self-neglect may become evident. This can take the form of failing to:

- Properly eat
- Take medications
- Keep appointments with health care providers
- Perform or obtain necessary treatments
- Maintain a clean, safe home

Family members who do not live in the same household with the older adult may not be aware of the situation. When self-neglect is suspected or confirmed, the nurse should urge the older person to discuss the need for help with family members or to grant permission for the nurse to contact the closest family member to discuss the situation.

Today's families are assisting with more complex issues and care for their older relatives than ever before, and doing so for a longer period of time. The increasing demands on families, changes in family structures, and impact of greater number of women employed outside the home heighten the challenges family members have in providing assistance.

Even if they are unable to provide regular caregiving assistance, family members serve an important role in the lives of their older relatives by providing emotional support, social contact, occasional assistance, and crisis management. The security of knowing they can count on their families if needed, and the satisfaction derived from remaining connected to their loved ones can contribute to a sense of satisfaction for older adults and their families.

16

Medication Use

The high prevalence of chronic conditions among older adults contributes to them using a significant number and wide range of medications. While medications enable older persons to survive conditions that were fatal to earlier generations and enjoy a high quality of life, they also carry risks that can cause significant problems. Nurses play an important role in ensuring medications produce more benefit than complications.

Objectives

In this chapter you will learn to:

1. List differences in pharmacokinetics and pharmacodynamics in older adults
2. Describe risks associated with medication use in older adults
3. Describe nursing considerations when older adults use:
   - Analgesics
   - Antacids
   - Antibiotics

- Antibiotics
- Antidiabetic drugs
- Antihypertensive drugs
- Cholesterol-lowering drugs
- Cognitive enhancing drugs for dementia
- Digoxin
- Diuretics
- Laxatives
- Nonsteroidal anti-inflammatory drugs (NSAIDs)
- Psychoactive drugs
4. List general nursing considerations with drug use in older adults

=== *FAST FACTS in a NUTSHELL*

> *The most commonly used medications among older adults are cardiovascular agents, antihypertensives, analgesics, antiarthritic agents, sedatives, tranquilizers, laxatives, and antacids.*

PHARMACOKINETICS AND PHARMACODYNAMICS IN LATE LIFE

Phamacokinetics refers to the way in which drugs behave in the body—their absorption, distribution, metabolism, and excretion. Aging has an impact on pharmacokinetics:

- *Absorption:* Reductions in muscle mass and subcutaneous tissue can affect the absorption of injected medications. Suppositories can take longer to absorb due to reduced circulation to the lower bowel. Absorption also can be affected by diseases common in older adults that increase gastric pH, reduce cardiac output and circulation, and decrease metabolism. Maintaining a normal body temperature, exercising, consuming adequate fluids, and using the gluteus maximus rather than arms for injections are among the factors that can promote absorption.

======================= *FAST FACTS in a NUTSHELL*

Biological half-life refers to the time required for half of a drug dose to be excreted from the body. Age-related changes can extend the biological half-life of many drugs by as much as 40% and lead to serious adverse effects. Drugs that are at high risk of being affected by this include antibiotics, barbiturates, cimetidine, digoxin, and salicylates.

- *Distribution:* Changes in circulation, body temperature, membrane permeability, and tissue structure can affect drug distribution. For example, older adults may have reduced serum albumin levels. If several protein-bound drugs (e.g., acetazolamide, amitriptyline, cefazolin, chlordiazepoxide, chlorpromazine, cloxacillin, digitoxin, furosemide, hydralazine, nortriptyline, phenylbutazone, phenytoin, propranolol, rifampin, salicylates, spironolactone, sulfisoxazole, and warfarin) are administered together, they can compete for the same protein molecules and displace each other, thereby reducing the effectiveness of the displaced drugs.
- *Metabolism:* Conditions that older adults frequently experience that can affect mobility, fluid intake, and body temperature can compound the reduced basal metabolic rate that is common in late life and, consequently, decrease drug metabolism. This can cause drugs to accumulate to toxic levels and adverse reactions to develop. Drugs that require enzymatic activity can be metabolized poorly due to the reduced secretion of some enzymes that occurs with age. The liver experiences a decrease in size, function, and hepatic blood flow with age; this can particularly affect the metabolism of antibiotics, cimetidine, chlordiazepoxide, digoxin, lithium, meperidine, nortriptyline, and quinidine.
- *Excretion:* With age, nephrons decrease in number and many of the remaining ones are nonfunctional. Reduced cardiac function results in decreased blood flow to the kidneys; glomerular filtration rate and tubular reabsorption are reduced. These factors contribute to drugs taking longer to be eliminated from the body.

FAST FACTS in a NUTSHELL

Older adults frequently will have a more profound response to drugs that affect the central nervous system (CNS). This is due to age-related decline in CNS function and increased pharmacodynamic sensitivity to some of the drugs that act upon this system.

Pharmacodynamics refers to the biologic and therapeutic effects of the drugs on the body. The most significant difference in the way drugs behave in the body is that older adults can have increased sensitivity to the drug's effects. This is particularly true of drugs with anticholinergic effects, such as tricyclic antidepressants, atropine-containing antiparkinsonian drugs, some antipsychotics, and many over-the-counter cold remedies. Increased drowsiness, urinary retention, constipation, orthostatic hypotension, and blurred vision are among the reactions that can occur. As reactions can vary and change with continued aging, the effects of drugs need to be assessed regularly.

FAST FACTS in a NUTSHELL

When new symptoms are identified in older individuals, the relationship of them to medications being used should be considered as part of the assessment.

RISKS

The effects of aging on pharmacokinetics and pharmacodynamics heighten the risk for adverse reactions to drugs in older adults. Careful attention is needed to detect adverse reactions because they could:

- Occur from a medication that has been used over a long period without any problem
- Produce signs and symptoms that differ from those that would appear in a younger adult
- Develop after the drug has been discontinued due to a sufficient amount of the drug still circulating in the body

Altered mental status, such as a delirium, is often an early sign of an adverse reaction. This is a particular risk in drugs that affect cerebral circulation, blood glucose levels, body temperature, and fluid and electrolyte balance. Deliriums can be difficult to detect in persons who have a dementia, and adverse drug reactions can easily be missed for this reason. Those who know these patients best should be taught to report even subtle changes in behavior and activity levels to the health care providers as they may detect mental status changes before those who are less frequently in contact with these patients.

A group of drugs that should be avoided for use in older adults due to their high risk for adverse reactions has been developed by Dr. Mark Beers and other experts. Known as the Beers Criteria for Potentially Inappropriate Medication Use in Older Adults, this document offers a list of drugs for which strong evidence exists supporting the recommendation to avoid usage of these drugs in the older population. Table 16.1 lists the drugs that are included

---

TABLE 16.1 Inappropriate Drugs to Use in Older Adults From Beers List

The following drugs are identified as having a high risk for adverse reactions in older adults:

First-generation antihistamines (as single agent or as part of combination products):
> brompheniramine, carbinoxamine, chlorpheniramine, clemastine, cyproheptadine, dexbrompheniramine, dexchlorpheniramine, diphenhydramine (oral), doxylamine, hydroxyzine, promethazine, triprolidine

Antiparkinsonian agents:
> benztropine (oral), trihexyphenidyl

Antispasmodics:
> belladonna alkaloids, clidinium-chlordiazepoxide, dicyclomine, hyoscyamine, propantheline scopolamine

Antihrombotics:
> dipyridamole, oral short-acting, ticlopidine

(continued)

TABLE 16.1 (Continued)

Anti-infective:
nitrofurantoin

Cardiovascular:
disopyramide
dronedarone
digoxin >0.125 mg/day
nifedipine, immediate release,
spironolactone >25 mg/day
alpha-1 blockers: doxazosin, prazosin, terazosin
alpha blockers, central: clonidine, guanabenz, guanfacine,
methyldopa, reserpine (>0.1 mg/day)
antiarrhythmic drugs (Class Ia, Ic, III): amiodarone, dofetilide,
  dronedarone, flecainide, Ibutilide, procainamide, propafenone,
  quinidine, sotalol

Central nervous system:
Tertiary TCAs, alone or in combination: amitriptyline, chlordiazepoxide-
  amitriptyline, clomipramine, doxepin >6 mg/day, imipramine,
  perphenazine-amitriptyline, trimipramine
Antipsychotics, first- (conventional) and second- (atypical) generation;
  thioridazine, mesoridazine
Barbiturates, amobarbital, butabarbital, butalbital, mephobarbital,
  pentobarbital, phenobarbital, secobarbital
Benzodiazepines: Short- and intermediate-acting: alprazolam,
  estazolam, lorazepam, oxazepam, temazepam, triazolam. Long-
  acting: chlorazepate, chlordiazepoxide, chlordiazepoxide-
  amitriptyline, clidinium-chlordiazepoxide, clonazepam, diazepam,
  flurazepam, quazepam
Chloral hydrate
Meprobamate
Nonbenzodiazepine hypnotics: eszopiclone, zolpidem, zaleplon
Ergot mesylates, isoxsuprine

Endocrine: Androgens: methyltestosterone, testosterone; desiccated
thyroid; estrogens with or without progestins; growth hormone;
insulin, sliding scale; megestrol; sulfonylureas (long-duration):
chlorpropamide, glyburide

Gastrointestinal:
metoclopramide
mineral oil, given orally
trimethobenzamide

(continued)

TABLE 16.1 (*Continued*)

Pain medications:
   meperidine
   Non–COX-selective NSAIDs, oral: aspirin >325 mg/day, diclofenac,
     diflunisal, etodolac, fenoprofen, ibuprofen, ketoprofen,
     meclofenamate, mefenamic acid, meloxicam, nabumetone,
     naproxen, oxaprozin, piroxicam, sulindac, tolmetin
   indomethacin, ketorolac, includes parenteral pentazocine
   Skeletal muscle relaxants: carisoprodol, chlorzoxazone,
     cyclobenzaprine, metaxalone, methocarbamol, orphenadrine

Adapted from The American Geriatrics Society 2012 Beers Criteria Update Expert Panel (2012). The American Geriatrics Society Updated Beers Criteria for Potentially Inappropriate Medication Use in Older Adults, *Journal of the American Geriatrics Society, 60*(4): 616–631.

on this list. The Beers Criteria Update Expert Panel also has identified drugs that are inappropriate to use when older adults have specific conditions due to the increased potential for adverse reactions (Table 16.2).

When assessing older adults, the nurse needs to be alert to the use of these medications when reviewing the drugs being used. If the use of these drugs is detected, the ongoing risk and benefit to the individual patient should be discussed with the prescribing physician.

CONSIDERATIONS WITH SELECTED DRUGS

It is essential that nurses understand the intended action, dosage range, side effects, adverse effects, and potential interactions with the drugs administered to older patients and ensure older adults and their caregivers who administer medications independently understand this information. This section will highlight specific age-related concerns related to the major drug groups used in the older population. To obtain a comprehensive review of medications, consult a current drug reference.

TABLE 16.2 Drugs to Avoid in the Presence of Specific Conditions Due to Increased Risk for Adverse Outcomes

Condition	Drugs to Avoid
Heart failure	NSAIDs and COX-2 inhibitors Pioglitazone, rosiglitazone Cilostazol Dronedarone
Delirium	Anticholinergics Benzodiazepines Chlorpromazine Corticosteroids H2-receptor antagonist Meperidine Sedative hypnotics Thioridazine
Dementia	Anticholinergics Benzodiazepines H2-receptor antagonists Zolpidem Antipsychotics
Parkinson's disease	All antipsychotics (except for quetiapine and clozapine) Antiemetics
Urinary incontinence (women)	Estrogen (oral and transdermal)
Stress or mixed urinary incontinence	Alpha-blockers
Chronic constipation	Oral antimuscarinics for urinary incontinence Nondihydropyridine CCB First-generation antihistamines as single agents or part of combination products Anticholinergics/antispasmodics
Insomnia	Oral decongestants Stimulants Theobromines
History of fractures or falls	Anticonvulsants Antipsychotics Benzodiazepines Nonbenzodiazepine hypnotics TCAs/SSRIs

Adapted from The American Geriatrics Society 2012 Beers Criteria Update Expert Panel (2012). American Geriatrics Society Beers Criteria for Potentially Inappropriate Medication Use in Older Adults Due to Drug–Disease or Drug–Syndrome Interactions That May Exacerbate the Disease or Syndrome, *Journal of the American Geriatrics Society*, 60(4): 616–631.

Analgesics

The high prevalence of conditions that cause pain in older adults causes analgesics to be a frequently used group of drugs. As these drugs carry risks to older persons, alternative pain relief measures should be considered, such as the application of heat, massage, relaxation exercises, acupressure, and diversional activities. When alternative measures are not effective in controlling pain, analgesics should be started with the weakest form at the lowest dosage. For persons with conditions that cause chronic pain, administering the analgesic on a regular schedule will help to maintain a constant level in the blood.

Aspirin

Older adults are high users of aspirin due to it being an effective, inexpensive pain reliever. They also are highly sensitive to aspirin's effects and are more likely to experience side effects, including serious ones such as gastrointestinal bleeding. Buffered or enteric-coated tablets and taking aspirin on a full stomach can reduce gastrointestinal irritation and bleeding. Aspirin consumption should be questioned when an older adult is found to have iron-deficiency anemia. Persons with reduced renal function can develop CNS disturbances; symptoms that could be associated with this include delirium, dizziness, tinnitus, and impaired hearing. The Beers Criteria recommends that aspirin not be consumed in amounts greater than 325 mg per day (Table 16.1). Observe for signs of salicylate toxicity, including dizziness, vomiting, tinnitus, hearing loss, sweating, fever, confusion, burning in the mouth and throat, convulsions, and coma. Be alert to potential drug-drug interactions:

- Aspirin can increase the effects of oral anticoagulants, oral antidiabetics, cortisone-like drugs, penicillins, and phenytoin, and decrease the effects of probenecid, spironolactone, and sulfinpyrazone
- The effects of aspirin can be increased by large doses of vitamin C, and decreased by antacids, phenobarbital, propranolol, and reserpine

FAST FACTS in a NUTSHELL

Aspirin can inhibit the kidney's excretion of uric acid and should be avoided in persons with gout or renal disease.

Acetaminophen

Acetaminophen is another popular analgesic due to its effectiveness in relieving mild to moderate pain. This drug can alter blood glucose levels, necessitating close monitoring when used in persons with diabetes. Doses exceeding 4,000 mg daily over a long period of time can cause irreversible liver damage; sometimes liver enzymes can become elevated with long-term use at lower dosages. For this reason, dosages may need to be adjusted for persons with altered liver function. Persons with renal or liver disease have a high risk for developing serious side effects. The effects of acetaminophen can be decreased by phenobarbital.

Opioids

The increased risk for adverse effects requires that these drugs be used with caution in older adults. Typically, the short-acting opioids are used for mild to moderate pain prior to initiating use of the long-acting opioids. Meperdine is viewed as an inappropriate drug for older adults due to its high risk for toxicity.

Antacids

Age-related changes to the gastrointestinal system and a higher prevalence of food intolerances create an increased use of antacids in late life. Although a commonly used group of medications that are highly marketed to consumers, antacids are not drugs to be used casually.

There are risks associated with antacid use; for example:

- Sodium bicarbonate can cause hypernatremia and metabolic acidosis
- Sodium bicarbonate and magnesium-containing antacids can cause diarrhea, leading to fluid and electrolyte imbalances
- Calcium carbonate can result in hypercalcemia
- Long-term use of calcium-based antacids can cause constipation and renal problems
- Long-term use of aluminum hydroxide can cause hyper-phosphatemia

Based on these risks, nurses should ensure antacids are not used casually. When these drugs have been used for a long period of time there may be a need for an evaluation to determine if there is a more serious problem contributing to the symptoms. Bowel elimination should be assessed and monitored when antacids are being used regularly.

It is recommended that antacids not be administered within 2 hours of other medications, as antacids can interfere with the absorption of other drugs. Examples of potential interactions include:

- Magnesium hydroxide can increase the effects of dicumarol
- Aluminum hydroxide can increase the effects of pseudo-ephedrine
- Most antacids can decrease the effects of barbiturates, chlorpromazine, digoxin, iron preparations, isoniazid, oral anticoagulants, penicillin, phenytoin, phenylbutazone, salicylates, sulfonamides, tetracycline, and vitamins A and C

Antibiotics

Older adults are more susceptible to infections and have more serious consequences when infections develop. Therefore, antibiotics have an important role in treatment. As valuable as they are, antibiotics do have their own risks and problems associated with their use in the older population:

- Some bacteria have become resistant to antibiotics due to their overuse
- Oral thrush, colitis, and vaginitis can occur as secondary infections from antibiotic therapy, affecting comfort, intake, and general well-being
- Diarrhea, nausea, vomiting, anorexia, and allergic reactions can occur with the use of antibiotics
- Hearing loss and renal failure can occur with the use of parenteral vancomycin and aminoglycosides
- Fluoroquinolones increase the risk of hypo- and hyperglycemia and can cause prolonged QTC intervals
- There can be false results with urine testing for glucose when cephalosporins are used

When signs of infection are present, cultures should be taken to match the most appropriate antibiotic with the organism. Antibiotics should be administered on a regular schedule to maintain a constant blood level; this is an important part of patient teaching. Close observation for new infections is essential, as superinfections can develop, whereby a new infection develops from a different microorganism and is resistant to the antibiotic already being used. Antibiotics can interact with other drugs and create new challenges for the older patient. Therefore, a review of all medications being used by the patient is important. Interactions could include:

- *Penicillin:* Effects can be reduced when taken with other highly protein-bound drugs such as aspirin, phenytoin, valproate, aripiprazole, buspirone, clozapine. Penicillin also could reduce the effects of these drugs.

FAST FACTS in a NUTSHELL

The reduction in protein molecules with age reduces the available protein molecules to which medications can attach. When several protein-bound molecules are administered concurrently, they can compete for the fewer protein molecules, some may not bind, and, consequently, the therapeutic benefit of the unbound drugs will not be gained.

- *Ampicillin and carbenicillin:* Effects can be decreased by antacids, chloramphenicol, erythromycin, and tetracycline.
- *Doxycycline:* Effects can be decreased by aluminum-, calcium-, or magnesium-based laxatives, antacids, iron preparations, phenobarbital, and alcohol.
- *Sulfisoxazole:* Effects can be increased by aspirin, oxyphenbutazone, probenecid, sulfinpyrazone, and para-aminosalicylic acid. Sulfisoxazole can increase the effects of alcohol, oral anticoagulants, oral antidiabetic agents, methotrexate, and phenytoin.

Anticoagulants

Older adults with a history of thromboembolic disorders, heart attacks, strokes, and coronary disorders are often prescribed anticoagulants (e.g., coumadin) as a means to prevent both arterial and venous thrombosis. In addition, these drugs can be used for prophylaxis for older adults undergoing certain types of surgeries. Close monitoring of prothrombin time (PT)/international normalization ratio (INR) is required when older adults are using anticoagulants, as these drugs carry a high risk for causing bleeding in this population. In addition, signs of bleeding need to be observed for, and patients administering these drugs independently need to be taught to observe and report signs of bleeding. Vitamin K is an antidote for anticoagulants and should be readily available when these drugs are used.

FAST FACTS in a NUTSHELL

Heparin typically is used for rapid anticoagulation and warfarin (coumadin) for long-term use.

Many drugs can interact with anticoagulants resulting in serious effects:

- Anticoagulants can increase the effects of oral hypoglycemic agents and phenytoin, and decrease the effects of cyclosporine and phenytoin
- Anticoagulants' effects can be increased by acetaminophen, allopurinol, alteplase, amprenavir, androgens, aspirin and some

other NSAIDs, azithromycin, bismuth subsalicylate, some calcium channel blockers, capsaicin, broad spectrum antibiotics, chlorpromazine, colchicine, ethacrynic acid, mineral oil, phenylbutazone, phenytoin, probenecid, reserpine, thyroxine, tolbutamide, and tricyclic antidepressants

- Anticoagulant effects can be decreased by antacids, antithyroid agents, barbiturates, carbamazepine, chlorpromazine, cholestyramine, estrogens, rifampin, thiazide diuretics, and vitamin K
- Heparin's effects can be partially reduced by digoxin, antihistamines, nicotine, and tetracyclines

ANTIDIABETIC DRUGS

See Chapter 10, under discussion on diabetes mellitus.

ANTIHYPERTENSIVE DRUGS

See Chapter 3, under discussion on hypertension.

CHOLESTEROL-LOWERING DRUGS

FAST FACTS in a NUTSHELL

Direct-to-consumer marketing has increased awareness of the benefits of these drugs and caused patients with high cholesterol to request them from their physicians.

Although treatment goals vary depending on the profile of the individual, the primary objective of using these drugs to lower cholesterol is to reduce low-density lipoprotein (LDL) and raise high-density lipoprotein (HDL). The use of cholesterol-lowering medications has grown and these drugs have shown benefit in reducing cardiovascular events and mortality in older adults. Drugs in this group include:

- *Statins (HMG-CoA reductase inhibitors):* These often are used as an initial treatment and work by blocking the production of cholesterol in the liver. Examples include rosuvastatin (Crestor), atorvastatin (Lipitor), fluvastatin (Lescol), lovastatin (Mevacor), pravastatin (Pravachol), and simvastatin (Zocor). Combination statins also are used, such as Advicor, a combination of a statin and niacin, and Caduet, a combination of a statin (atorvastatin) and the antihypertensive amlodipine (Norvasc). As these drugs can impair liver function, liver function tests should be done prior to initiating therapy and at regular intervals thereafter. These drugs can cause myopathy and the breakdown of skeletal muscle, which can precipitate renal failure.

- *Bile-acid resins:* These drugs work inside the intestine, where they bind to bile and prevent it from being reabsorbed into the circulatory system. Examples include cholestyramine (Questran and Questran Light), colestipol (Colestid), and colesevelam (WelChol). The most common side effects are constipation, gas, and upset stomach. These drugs can interact with diuretics, beta-blockers, corticosteroids, thyroid hormones, digoxin, valproic acid, NSAIDs, sulfonylureas, and warfarin; consult with the physician and pharmacist as to the length of time to wait between the administration of these drugs and bile-acid resins.

- *Niacin:* In addition to dietary intake, niacin or nicotinic acid can be prescribed at high dosages to lower LDL and raise HDL cholesterol. Examples include Niacor, Niaspan, and Slo-niacin. The main side effects are flushing, itching, tingling, and headache; aspirin can reduce many of these symptoms. Niacin can interfere with glucose control and aggravate diabetes. It also can exacerbate gallbladder disease and gout.

- *Fibric acid derivatives:* The mechanism of action of these drugs is not fully clear, though they are thought to enhance the breakdown of triglyceride-rich particles, decrease the secretion of certain lipoproteins, and induce the synthesis of HDL. Examples include fenofibrate (Tricor), gemfibrozil (Lopid), and fenofibrate (Lofibra). Liver function tests and CBC should be evaluated prior to initiating therapy and on a regular basis thereafter.

- *Cholesterol absorption inhibitors*: These drugs inhibit the absorption of cholesterol in the intestines; ezetimibe (Zetia) is an example. Vytorin is a newer drug that is a combination of ezetimibe and the statin simvastatin.

FAST FACTS in a NUTSHELL

It is beneficial to instruct patients in nonpharmacologic measures to reduce cholesterol prior to the use of medications. These measures can include a heart-healthy diet, weight reduction, and exercise.

COGNITIVE-ENHANCING DRUGS FOR DEMENTIA

This group of drugs does not eliminate dementias, but, in some individuals, aids in maximizing existing cognitive function. They consist of:

- *Cholinesterase inhibitors:* donepezil (Aricept), galantamine (Razadyne), rivastigmine tartrate (Exelon), tacrine (Cognex)
- *NMDA receptor antagonists:* memantine (Namenda).

Considerations with the use of these drugs include:

- A good baseline of physical and mental function should be done prior to initiating therapy and periodically thereafter.
- Side effects need to be observed for and will most commonly include: nausea, vomiting, diarrhea, anorexia, weight loss, urinary frequency, muscle cramps, joint pain, swelling or stiffness, fatigue, drowsiness, headache, dizziness, nervousness, depression, confusion, changes in behavior, abnormal dreams, difficulty falling asleep or staying asleep, discoloration or bruising of the skin, and red, scaling, itchy skin.
- Risks of using cholinesterase inhibitors in persons with cardiac conduction disorders or who are using medications that affect heart rate should be evaluated by the physician, as changes in conduction can occur.

- Galantamine is best taken with food; tacrine is best taken on an empty stomach.
- Regular liver function tests should be performed on individuals using tacrine.
- These drugs should not be abruptly discontinued.

DIGOXIN

Digoxin improves circulation by increasing the force of myocardial contraction through direct action on the heart muscle. It is used to treat congestive heart failure, atrial flutter fibrillation, supraventricular tachycardia, and extrasystoles.

The biological half-life of digoxin can be prolonged in some older persons, which will increase their risk for digitalis toxicity. The risk of toxicity is increased when digoxin is taken with cortisone, diuretics, parenteral calcium reserpine, and thyroid preparations. Signs of toxicity include bradycardia, diarrhea, anorexia, nausea, vomiting, abdominal pain, delirium, agitation, hallucinations, headache, restlessness, insomnia, nightmares, aphasia, ataxia, muscle weakness and pain, cardiac arrhythmias, and high serum drug levels. Serum levels of the drug should be monitored.

FAST FACTS in a NUTSHELL

Digitalis toxicity can occur in the presence of normal serum levels of the drug, which emphasizes the need to observe for clinical signs of toxicity.

It is important to consider the following when digoxin is used:

- Do not exceed a daily dose of 0.125 mg unless the physician has intentionally ordered a higher dose to control atrial arrhythmia and ventricular rate.
- Always check pulse for rate, rhythm, and regularity prior to administering digoxin.
- For individuals who are administering the medication independently, instruct them and their caregivers to check

the pulse prior to administration. Also provide them with information about digitalis toxicity and instruct them to notify their health care provider if any of the signs are present.

- Ensure the patient consumes potassium-rich foods regularly, as hypokalemia will increase susceptibility to toxicity. Ensure that the serum potassium is evaluated regularly.
- Use digoxin with caution in patients with impaired renal function.
- Be alert to interactions that digoxin may have with other drugs; for example, the effects of digoxin can be:
  - Increased by alprazolam, amphotericin, benzodiazepines, carvedilol, cyclosporine, erythromycin, ethacrynic acid, fluoxetine, guanethidine, ibuprofen, indomethacin, phenytoin, propranolol, quinidine, tetracyclines, tolbutamide, trazodone, trimethoprim, and verapamil
  - Decreased by antacids, cholestyramine, kaolin-pectin, laxatives, neomycin, phenobarbital, phenylbutazone, and rifampin

DIURETICS

Diuretics are commonly used with older persons who have hypertension, congestive heart failure, and other cardiovascular disorders. There are several types that work in different ways:

- *Thiazides* (e.g., include chlorothiazide, hydrochlorothiazide, metolazone) inhibit sodium reabsorption in the cortical diluting site of the ascending loop of Henle and increase the excretion of chloride and potassium.
- *Loop diuretics* (e.g., bumetanide, ethacrynic acid, furosemide) inhibit reabsorption of sodium and chloride at the proximal portion of the ascending loop of Henle.
- *Potassium-sparing diuretics* (e.g., amiloride, spironolactone, triamterene) antagonize aldosterone in the distal tubule, causing water and sodium, but not potassium, to be excreted.

Older adults are at high risk of becoming dehydrated and diuretics can heighten this risk. Patients may mistakenly think that if they are taking a medication to eliminate fluid, they should consume less fluid. Part of patient teaching includes the importance of a good fluid intake. Other measures to consider include:

- Provide necessary assistance with toileting as frequent voiding will occur.
- Monitor intake and output.
- Ensure serum electrolytes, glucose, and BUN are evaluated periodically.
- As postural hypotension sometimes occurs during diuretic therapy, advise the patient to change positions slowly.
- Recognize and promptly report signs of fluid and electrolyte imbalance, such as dry oral cavity, confusion, thirst, weakness, lethargy, drowsiness, restlessness, muscle cramps, muscular fatigue, hypotension, reduced urinary output, slow pulse, and GI disturbances. Teach these signs to the patient and the caregivers.
- Diuretics can raise blood glucose in persons with diabetes and worsen existing liver disease, renal disease, gout, and pancreatitis. Close monitoring is essential.
- Be alert to interactions:
  - Diuretics can increase the effects of antihypertensives.
  - Diuretics can decrease the effects of allopurinol, digoxin, oral anticoagulants, antidiabetic agents, and probenecid.
  - The effects of diuretics can be increased by analgesics and barbiturates.
  - The effects of diuretics can be decreased by cholestyramine and large quantities of aspirin (administer these drugs at least 1 hour before).

FAST FACTS in a NUTSHELL

Diuretics are usually best administered in the morning so that their peak effect won't interrupt sleep.

LAXATIVES

The reduced peristalsis that occurs with age, diets that lack sufficient fiber, inactivity, and constipating medications contribute to a high use of laxatives among older adults. As this is a common problem, questions about bowel elimination need to be a routine part of every assessment. If constipation is identified as a problem, questions should be asked about its onset, pattern, and management.

FAST FACTS in a NUTSHELL

It is important to learn about factors that may have contributed to constipation, not only to find alternatives to laxative use, but also to identify diseases that require attention.

[Clinical Snapshot]

Mr. C started using cholestyramine about 6 weeks ago and is experiencing constipation (one of the side effects of the drug). When asking Mr. C about symptoms in general, the nurse learns that due to indigestion problems, Mr. C also changed his diet over the past 2 months and has been consuming more cream-based soups and cheeses. Whereas recommendations for the inclusion of more high-fiber foods may be effective in improving the situation for the patient using cholestyramine, Mr. C's constipation and indigestion problems may be associated with an undiagnosed GI disorder that requires evaluation, and this should be explored prior to making the dietary recommendations.

When other measures are ineffective in preventing and correcting constipation, a laxative may be needed. Laxatives should be selected based on the type of problem and desired action; they can include:

- *Stool softeners* (e.g., docusate sodium), act by collecting fluid in the stool, which makes the mass softer and easier to move. They do not stimulate peristalsis; they take effect in 24 to 48 hours.
- *Bulk formers* (e.g., methylcellulose), which absorb fluid in the intestines and create extra bulk, that distends the intestines and increases peristalsis. They usually take 12 to 24 hours to

take effect. They need to be mixed with large amounts of water. These compounds are contraindicated when there is any indication of intestinal obstruction.

- *Stimulants* (e.g., cascara sagrada), irritate the smooth muscle of the intestines and pull fluid into the colon, causing peristalsis. They take effect in 6 to 10 hours. They can cause intestinal cramps and excessive fluid evacuation.
- *Hyperosmolars* (e.g., glycerin) pull fluid into the colon, causing bowel distension, which increases peristalsis. These take effect within 1 to 3 hours. They should not be used when there is the risk of fecal impaction.
- *Lubricants* (e.g., mineral oil), which coat fecal material to facilitate its passage. They take effect in 6 to 8 hours. These compounds are not recommended for older adults, as they can cause serious problems if aspirated during administration, and, if used on a long-term basis, can cause a depletion of fat-soluble vitamins (A,D, K, and E).

Patients need to understand that laxatives are medications that can produce problems (e.g., diarrhea, vitamin depletion) and need to be use with care. Patients should be encouraged to include foods in their diets that could stimulate bowel movements, increase activity, and consume a good fluid intake.

NONSTEROIDAL ANTI-INFLAMMATORY DRUGS (NSAIDs)

When lower-risk analgesics such as acetaminophen are ineffective in managing mild to moderate pain and inflammation, NSAIDs may be used. Examples of NSAIDs include cyclooxygenase-II (COX-2) inhibitors, diclofenac, diflunisal, flurbiprofen, indomethacin, meclofenamate, naproxen, piroxicam, salicylates, and tolmetin. Oxyphenbutazone and phenylbutazone are extremely potent NSAIDs and carry a high risk of adverse effects for older adults.

NSAIDs have a smaller therapeutic window and can easily accumulate to toxic levels. Side effects indicating problems include gastrointestinal disturbances, impaired hearing, and signs of CNS disturbances. Blood levels should be obtained regularly.

FAST FACTS in a NUTSHELL

Cerecoxib (Celebrex) is a COX-2 inhibitor that is used by many people due to its effectiveness in managing arthritis pain. However, in older adults it carries the serious and even fatal risks for cardiovascular thrombotic events, myocardial infarction, and stroke, as well as an increased risk of GI adverse events including bleeding, ulceration, and perforation of the stomach or intestines. It is recommended that it be used at the lowest effective dose for the shortest possible time.

Nurses should ensure precautions are taken when NSAIDs are used, including:

- Advising patients to take these drugs with food or a glass of milk, unless contraindicated, to reduce GI irritation.
- Closely observing for side effects, such as GI symptoms, impaired hearing, and indications of CNS disturbances, delirium, and a worsening of any existing renal disease, hypertension, and heart failure.
- Ensuring blood evaluations are done regularly.
- Avoiding the use of oxyphenbutazone and phenylbutazone on a long-term basis and in patients with blood disorders; dementia; GI ulcers; glaucoma; or cardiac, renal, liver, or thyroid disease.
- Preventing interactions:
  - NSAIDs can increase the effects of oral anticoagulants, insulin, oral antidiabetic drugs, cyclosporine, lithium, penicillin, phenytoin, and sulfa drugs.
  - NSAIDs can decrease the effects of diuretics and beta blockers.

PSYCHOACTIVE DRUGS

While not a normal outcome of aging, mental health conditions do affect a significant number of older adults, and persons over age 85 years have a suicide rate that is more than twice the national average. Anxiety and depression often go unreported or are missed by health care providers; untreated, these conditions threaten the quality of life and the self-care independence. While psychoactive drugs can address these problems, they do carry an increased risk for adverse events in older persons. They need to be prescribed with care and monitored closely when they are used.

FAST FACTS in a NUTSHELL

Psychoactive drugs have a prolonged biological half-life in older adults; therefore, they will remain in the body longer and accumulate to toxic levels more easily. This can result in episodes of delirium, falls, and other adverse incidents. These drugs need to be used cautiously and closely monitored in older individuals.

ANTIANXIETY DRUGS (ANXIOLYTICS)

Reduced finances, new health conditions, deaths of loved ones, relocation, and retirement are among the problems that offer legitimate reason for some anxiety among older adults.

FAST FACTS in a NUTSHELL

Antianxiety medications should only be used when there is generalized anxiety disorder, panic disorder, anxiety that accompanies another psychiatric disorder, sleep disorder, significant anxiety in response to a situational trigger, or delirium, dementia, and other cognitive disorders with associated behaviors that are well documented, persistent, not due to preventable or correctable reasons, and create such distress or dysfunction to make the person a risk to self or others (American Psychiatric Association, 2013).

If evaluation supports that an antianxiety medication is warranted, the patient needs to be prescribed carefully. Options used include:

- *Beta-blockers:* These drugs temper the effects of adrenaline and lower blood pressure, which can provide relief of anxiety.

They carry the risk of causing depression and are contraindicated for long-term use.

- *Benzodiazepines:* Although a popular class of tranquilizer that are effective for anxiety and viewed as preferable to barbiturates for older adults, these drugs do carry risks for older adults including depression, psychological dependence, delirium, and falls.
- *Antidepressants:* In addition to being an effective drug to treat depression, selective serotonin reuptake inhibitors (SSRIs) are effective in the treatment of chronic anxiety. Common side effects include insomnia, dry mouth, fatigue, gastric upset, dizziness, restlessness, tremors, and, in some cases, a worsening of anxiety.
- *Buspirone:* This drug does not produce the muscle relaxant and sedation effects of benzodiazepines.

FAST FACTS in a NUTSHELL

Barbiturates and benzodiazepines are included on the Beers List of Drugs That Are Inappropriate to Use for Older Adults.

Nursing considerations when antianxiety medications are used include:

- Ensure nonpharmacologic measures to reduce anxiety have been attempted before seeking an antianxiety drug for the patient.
- Alert patients to the fact that several days of administration of these drugs may be needed before effects are noted, and effects can still be present days after these drugs are discontinued.
- As these drugs can dull responses, caution the patient against driving, climbing ladders, and changing positions quickly until adjustment to the drug has been made.
- Abdominal cramping can occur from these drugs; monitor nutritional status.
- Constipation can occur as a side effect. Encourage the patient to increase fiber and other foods in the diet that can enhance bowel elimination.

- Caffeine should be limited and alcohol avoided when using these drugs.
- Be alert to interactions; antianxiety drugs can interact with:
  - Anticonvulsants
  - Antidepressants
  - Diazepam
  - Digoxin
  - Diltiazem
  - Erythromycin
  - Grapefruit juice
  - Haloperidol
  - Levodopa
  - Nefazodone
  - Rifampin
  - Ritonavir
  - Some antifungal medicines (e.g., itraconazole, ketoconazole, and voriconazole)
  - Verapamil
  - Warfarin

ANTIDEPRESSANTS

As depression is the major psychiatric diagnosis among older adults, it is not uncommon to find many older persons using antidepressants. There are several types of antidepressants used with older adults, including:

- Tetracyclic/alpha-adrenoceptors (e.g., mirtazapine)
- Cyclic antidepressants (e.g., amoxapine, imipramine, nortriptyline)
- Dopamine-reuptake blocking compounds (e.g., bupropion)
- Serotonin antagonists/modulators (5-HT 2, e.g., nefazodone, trazodone)
- Selective serotonin-norepinephrine reuptake inhibitors (SNRIs, e.g., duloxetine, venlafaxine)
- Selective serotonin reuptake inhibitors (SSRIs, e.g., citalopram, escitalopram, fluoxetine, fluvoxamine, paroxetine, sertraline) and tricyclic antidepressants (TCAs)

Of the antidepressants that could be selected, the SSRIs tend to be safer, better tolerated and effective in older adults, and typically do not cause cardiotoxicity, orthostatic hypotension, or anticholinergic effects as do tricyclic antidepressants. They are not without their risks, however. Because they are metabolized in the liver and some of the drugs in this group are highly bound to plasma protein, they can interact with other drugs that are metabolized in the liver or that are protein bound. The risk of GI bleeding is high when SSRIs are taken with aspirin or NSAIDs.

Nursing considerations with the use of antidepressants include:

- Perform a comprehensive assessment to identify factors that contribute to the depression. For example, if depression is caused by the inability to pay a bill, financial aid rather than medication is more beneficial.
- Support the use of other therapies to complement drug therapy.
- Provide education to the patient regarding facts about antidepressant therapy, which includes points such as:
  - Several weeks of therapy may be needed before results may be seen; it could take several months before the full results of the drug's effectiveness are realized
  - The drug needs to be taken on a regular schedule and as prescribed
  - Side effects may develop, including diaphoresis, urinary retention, indigestion, constipation, hypotension, blurred vision, difficulty voiding, increased appetite, weight gain, photosensitivity, and fluctuating blood glucose levels
  - Dry mouth may occur, which can be improved by sugarless mints, ice chips, or a saliva substitute
  - Dizziness and drowsiness may occur, so be careful when changing positions; driving should be avoided until the effects are known and stabilized
  - Do not stop taking the drug abruptly
  - Contact your health care provider if your symptoms worsen or if you have thoughts of harming yourself
- Be alert to interactions:
  - Antidepressants can increase the effects of anticoagulants, atropine-like drugs, antihistamines, sedatives, tranquilizers, narcotics, and levodopa

- Antidepressants can decrease the effects of clonidine, phenytoin, and various antihypertensives
- Alcohol and thiazide diuretics can increase the effects of antidepressants

ANTIPSYCHOTICS

Antipsychotic medications have been used as a means to manage behaviors in persons with delirium, agitation, and psychosis due to Alzheimer's disease and schizophrenia. Although these drugs have been effective in controlling symptoms sufficiently to enable patients to function and be cared for, they have come under considerable scrutiny in recent years as concern about their serious adverse effects has grown.

The major categories of antipsychotics are:

- *First-generation (conventional) agents:* chlorpromazine, flumezapine, haloperidol, loxapine, mesoridazine, promazine, thioridazine, thiothixene, trifluoperazine, triflupromazine
- *Second-generation (atypical) agents:* aripiprazole, clozapine, olanzapine, quetiapine, risperidone, ziprasidone

The atypical antipsychotics, which once were used with greater confidence than the conventional ones, have been found to produce serious effects.

=========== *FAST FACTS in a NUTSHELL*

After identifying that the treatment of behavioral disorders in older patients with dementia with atypical or second-generation antipsychotic medications was associated with increased cerebrovascular adverse events and mortality, the Food and Drug Administration (FDA) issued a black box warning, stating that these drugs should only be used for the treatment of schizophrenia and not for behavioral disturbances associated with dementias (FDA, 2005).

Nursing considerations related to antipsychotic drug use include:

- Options to control symptoms and behaviors other than drugs should be considered before antipsychotic drugs are prescribed.
- The use of antipsychotic medications for behavioral symptoms should be part of a comprehensive plan for behavioral health and management.
- Ensure the patient has a comprehensive assessment prior to using an antipsychotic.
- Older adults should be started on the lowest possible dosage of the drug and observed for response.
- Because these drugs have hypotensive and sedative effects, active measures to prevent falls in patients using antipsychotics are needed.
- These drugs have a high risk for producing *anticholinergic effects and extrapyramidal* symptoms.

Observe for:

  - *Anticholinergic symptoms:* dry mouth, constipation, urinary retention, blurred vision, insomnia, restlessness, fever, confusion, disorientation, hallucinations, agitation, picking behavior.
  - *Extrapyramidal symptoms:* tardive dyskinesia, parkinsonism, akinesia, dystonia.

- Constipation is a common side effect of antipsychotics; preventive measures should be implemented when these drugs are used.
- Individuals can vary in their response to antipsychotics, and response to an antipsychotic can change in the same individual over time. Ongoing monitoring is essential.
- Observe for *neuroleptic malignant syndrome* (NMS), a rare but serious complication associated with the use of antipsychotics that results from drug-induced decreased dopaminergic activity (National Institute of Neurological Disorders & Stroke, National Institutes of Health, 2013). It usually develops within the first few weeks of therapy, although it can occur at any time during therapy. Signs include: high fever, sweating, muscle rigidity, and an unstable blood pressure among others. This occurs more frequently in patients with a pre-existing neurological condition, the presence of agitation or dehydration,

and with high doses of antipsychotics. This is a serious condition that can be fatal if not treated early; usually intensive care treatment is needed.

- These drugs should not be discontinued abruptly.
- Be alert to interactions:
  - Antipsychotics can increase the effects of sedatives and antihypertensives, and decrease the effects of levodopa
  - The effects of antipsychotics can be reduced by anticholinergic drugs, phenytoin, and antacids

FAST FACTS in a NUTSHELL

Antipsychotic medications should not be used merely for the control of behaviors. Using them solely for this reason could be considered a form of chemical restraint.

HYPNOTICS

FAST FACTS in a NUTSHELL

Sedatives are drugs that slow activity and have a calming effect. At higher doses these same drugs induce sleep and are considered hypnotics.

Sleep disturbances are common among older adults. At one time, benzodiazepines were widely prescribed hypnotics, but their high incidence of adverse effects has caused them to now be contraindicated. Nonbenzodiazepines (e.g., eszopiclone, ramelteon, zaleplon, zolpidem) are now considered safer, although with the exception of eszopiclone, they are not approved for long-term use. The nonbenzodiazepines do have the risk for serious adverse effects, including falls, sleep walking, residual sedation, and memory and performance impairment.

Nursing considerations with the use of hypnotics in older adults include:

- Perform a comprehensive assessment when sleep disturbances are present. Factors contributing to sleep disturbances can include pain, insufficient daytime activity, nocturia, new environment, noisy environment, interruptions for treatments, and the effects of medications. If there are factors contributing to sleep disturbances, address them.

- Use nonpharmacologic means to relax patients and induce sleep, such as backrubs, warm milk, guided imagery, progressive relaxation, relaxing music, and aromatherapy with lavender.
- Encourage daytime activity and exercise.
- Control environmental noise and interruptions.
- Explore underlying fears, conflicts, and unresolved problems that may be contributing to sleeplessness.
- Monitor the ongoing effectiveness of the hypnotic. Some patients develop increasing tolerance after a month of use and find the hypnotic no longer beneficial.
- Be alert to interactions:
  - Hypnotics can increase the effects of oral anticoagulants, antihistamines, and analgesics, and decrease the effects of cortisone and cortisone-like drugs
  - Effects of sedatives and hypnotics can be increased by alcohol, antihistamines, and phenothiazines

GENERAL NURSING CONSIDERATIONS

Most older adults have health conditions that require medications. While beneficial in controlling symptoms and treating diseases, drugs do pose risks due to the different ways in which they behave in the older body, their potential to interact with each other, and the side effects and adverse reactions they cause. Nurses play a significant role in ensuring that older adults obtain greater benefit than risks from medications.

A review of all prescription and over-the-counter medications should be part of every assessment. When reviewing the medications, consideration should be given to:

- *The reason the drug is being used.* It could be that the original problem for which a drug was ordered has resolved, or a non-pharmacologic measure could substitute for the drug.
- *The appropriateness of the dosage.* Age-adjusted dosages are needed for many medications. In addition, as the individual

ages, the dose that was appropriate several years ago may be excessive today.

- *The appropriateness of administration.* If the patient or lay caregivers are administering medications, there should be a review of the manner in which they are taking the drugs (e.g., time, dosage, and adherence to any special instructions for administration).

FAST FACTS in a NUTSHELL

It is beneficial to review the patient's (or caregiver's) understanding of the purpose, use, schedule of administration, and related precautions of every drug administered, even for drugs used over a long period of time. It cannot be assumed that the patient has been adequately taught or remembers all instructions related to the drugs used.

- *Effects of the drug.* The effectiveness of the drug in bringing about the desired result needs to be assessed, in addition to any side effects or adverse reactions that may be present.
- *Potential interactions.* It is useful to inquire about all drugs, herbs, and nutritional supplements the patient is using to determine their potential for interactions.
- *Results of laboratory tests.* Records should be reviewed related to laboratory tests that are ordered to monitor blood levels of the drug. Abnormal results should be communicated to the prescribing health care provider.

By ensuring the ongoing effectiveness and safety of drug therapy, nurses can assist older adults in obtaining maximum therapeutic benefit from medications with minimal risks.

17

Legal Issues

Nursing in any specialty carries legal risks; in geriatric nursing the vulnerability of the population served and the complex clinical and psychosocial issues they present heighten these risks considerably. Challenges also arise due to the settings in which older adult are cared for. For example, in nursing homes, most direct care and contact that older adults have are with unlicensed personnel who have minimal training. Their inexperience and lack of preparation can cause situations in which the older person's rights are not respected or a change in status goes unrecognized and liability results. Older adults living independently in the community may fall victim to unscrupulous practices or not understand legal safeguards to protect themselves and their property. Special effort is needed to ensure the preferences of older adults are respected, they are not taken advantage of due to their condition, the care they receive complies with recognized standards, and that they have responsible agents acting on their behalf in the event that they are no longer able to make competent decisions.

Objectives

In this chapter you will learn to:

1. Differentiate public from private law
2. List items described in practice acts
3. Describe the meaning of and ways to minimize the risks associated with elder abuse
4. Describe common types of advance directives
5. Describe various types of guardianship that can be granted on an incompetent person's behalf
6. List the elements of informed consent
7. Describe when a do not resuscitate order is needed
8. Describe key points of HIPAA
9. List examples of restraints
10. Describe what is meant by and how to minimize risks associated with
    - Assault and battery
    - Defamation
    - False imprisonment
    - Incidents and accidents
    - Malpractice
    - Respondeat superior
    - Telephone orders

NURSING PRACTICE AND THE LAW

In addition to clinical information and skills, nurses must include an understanding of laws affecting nursing practice as part of their foundational knowledge. These laws can be specific to health care, such as Nurse Practice Acts, the Patient Self-Determination Act, and the Health Insurance Portability and Accountability Act (HIPAA); they can also involve issues that can affect interactions among people generally, such as assault, battery, and defamation.

Laws can be developed on the federal, state, and local levels. *Public laws* are those that involve relationships between the government and individuals, institutions, or businesses. Murder, rape, vehicle speeding, and standards for operating various business enterprises fall in this category. Regulations that govern the operation of health care facilities are an example of public law.

Private law addresses relationships between private parties, such as a business and an individual or two individuals. Malpractice and employment contracts are examples of this type of law.

Nurses are governed by practice acts, which are laws that describe:

- Educational requirements
- The scope of practice
- Licensure requirements
- Titles that are allowed to be used
- Consequences of not following the nursing law

There are practice acts specific to registered nurses, licensed practical nurses, nursing assistants, advanced practice nurses, and medication aides. These laws serve to protect the public. Each state has a nurse practice act that has been enacted by the state legislature that describes the scope of nursing practice in the specific state. When moving and practicing in another state, the nurse must apply for licensure in that state and abide by the nurse practice act of that state.

It is important for nurses to be familiar with the practice act governing their specific nursing license, as well as the practice acts of other nursing staff to whom tasks may be delegated. In addition to ensuring they stay within the legal scope of their own license, nurses must be sure not to delegate tasks to others that are beyond their scope of practice.

FAST FACTS in a NUTSHELL

The National Council of State Boards of Nursing's website contains contact information for every state's board of nursing, which can assist nurses in finding the nurse practice act in a specific state.

Liability refers to the legal responsibility that people carry for an act. A nurse can be liable for:

- Injuries resulting from not fulfilling an obligation
- Performing an act without following the accepted standard

- The wrongful or neglectful acts of other levels of nursing staff to whom the nurse delegates responsibilities
- Wrongful acts that the nurse commits to other employees

The remainder of this chapter reviews specific areas of liability and measures to reduce them.

PATIENT PROTECTION

Abuse

FAST FACTS in a NUTSHELL

The National Center for Elder Abuse estimates that 2.1 million older Americans are victims of elder abuse, neglect, or exploitation every year, and that for every case reported, as many as five cases go unreported (National Center for Elder Abuse, 2013).

Doing or threatening to do physical, psychological, financial, or sexual harm to a person is considered abuse. There are several major types of abuse that older adults can experience (National Center for Elder Abuse, 2013):

- Physical abuse
- Emotional abuse
- Sexual abuse
- Exploitation
- Neglect
- Abandonment

Older adults may be reluctant to admit to or report abuse. This can be due to:

- Fear that the abuser may become angry and inflict greater harm
- Dependency on the abuser

- Concern about the alternative if separated from the abuser
- Lack of physical or mental capacity to identify or report the abuse

For these reasons, nurses need to be alert to signs of possible abuse; these could include:

- Poor hygiene and grooming
- Failure to obtain necessary care or medications
- Unexplained bruises or injuries
- Malnutrition, dehydration, unexplained weight loss
- Odorous clothing
- Excoriation, bruises, or pain of genital area
- Reluctance to discuss problems
- Social withdrawal or isolation
- Unclean or unsafe living conditions
- Unexplained loss or mismanagement of funds
- Suspiciousness
- Depression

The law requires that all suspected or known abuse be reported; in fact, many states have laws that make it a crime not to report abuse. The reporting procedure varies based on state and setting. (See the Resources section for organizations that can provide information and assistance regarding elder abuse.)

Advance Directives

An advance directive is a legally binding document developed by a competent individual that expresses preferences about care for use at a future time if the person is no longer able to make his own decisions. Common types of advance directives include:

- *Durable power of attorney,* which allows the patient to designate a person (called a proxy decision maker, health care proxy, agent, surrogate, or attorney-in-fact) who will be responsible for communicating the patient's preferences if the patient is unable to do so
- *Living will,* which is a legal document stating the type of medical treatment that the patient would and would not want if he or she was incapable of expressing preferences

The Patient Self-Determination Act, enacted by Congress in 1990 and becoming effective in 1991, required that health care organizations had to:

- Inform patients of their right to make health care decisions and refuse treatments
- Ask patients if they had completed an advance directive
- Provide written information about their state's provisions for implementing advance directives
- Include documentation of patients' advance directives in their medical records
- Educate the staff and community about advance directives

This legislation requires that nurses ask patients about advance directives. Patients who have not developed an advance directive should be assisted in doing so if they are mentally competent. In nursing homes, federal regulations state that the patient has a right to a written description of the facility's policies to implement advance directive and applicable state law.

FAST FACTS in a NUTSHELL

All states and the District of Columbia have laws that require all adults to have living wills. States vary in the type of document used, scope, and conditions under which it is used, as well as their acceptance of advance directives written in other states.

The nurse plays an important role in inquiring about this document and facilitating discussions with patients about their desires. If the nurse identifies that the patient is uncomfortable with what has been expressed in the advance directive or wishes to change it, the patient should be assisted in doing so. A copy of the patient's advance directive should be included in the medical record and all members of the interdisciplinary team should be aware of and respect its contents.

Competency

People are considered competent to make their own decisions unless judged incompetent in a court of law. There are situations, however, when an older adult has not been declared incompetent by a judge but seems unable to make reasonable decisions. This is particularly true when the person has a cognitive impairment. At these times the person designated as the health care proxy (see Advance Directives discussion) will assume the decision-making responsibility. If a health care proxy has not been designated or there is concern among significant others in the patient's life about the named health care proxy, a petition can be filed with the probate court to determine competency and assign guardianship (conservatorship).

There are different types of guardianship that can be granted on the incompetent person's behalf:

- *Guardian of person:* the person has legal authority to refuse or consent to care and treatments for the patient
- *Guardian of property* (limited guardianship, conservatorship): the person is able to take care of financial matters and legal transactions for the patient, but not make decisions concerning medical treatment
- *Plenary guardianship* (committeeship): the person has legal authority and responsibility for decisions over patient's property and personal care and treatments

Guardianship differs from *power of attorney* in that competent individuals can use a power of attorney mechanism to appoint someone to make decisions for them. A *limited power of attorney* can be granted, which gives authorization to someone to make only specific decisions for the individual (e.g., to be able to sign contracts pertaining to financial matters). Usually, this power of attorney is discontinued if the individual granting it becomes incompetent. A mechanism for continuing the power of attorney in

FAST FACTS in a NUTSHELL

It is important to request copies of the power of attorney or guardianship documents when family members or other individuals claim to have power of attorney or guardianship for a patient, as they may be restricted in decisions they can make, have guardianship of property but not be able to make medical decisions, or not be honestly representing the situation.

the event of the onset of incompetency or to initiating it in the event that the individual becomes incompetent is to assign *durable power of attorney*. Patients who wish to assign power of attorney and families who want to obtain guardianship should be referred to an attorney to ensure that these procedures are done in a legally valid manner.

Consent

Written consent demonstrates that the patient authorizes the health care provider or organization (hospital, nursing home, assisted living community, home health agency, etc.) to perform specific procedures. Most agencies have a consent form that patients sign upon admission that authorizes the organization to perform routine and customary services, such as administering medications and bathing. Additional consent is needed for each procedure that exceeds basic care; this would include:

- Surgery
- Use of anesthesia
- Moderate- to high-risk diagnostic procedures
- Use of cobalt or radiation
- Electroshock therapy
- Experimental drugs or procedures
- Participation in research

Consent must be *informed* and the following will help to ensure that it is:

- Provide the patient with a full verbal and written description of the procedure, its name, its purpose, the steps that will occur, alternatives, consequences, possible side effects, and risks.
- Offer the description on a level and in a language that the patient can understand.
- The professional responsible for performing the procedure should obtain the consent from the patient. If that responsibility

is delegated, the person performing the procedure remains liable.

- If the patient has been determined to be legally incompetent, obtain written consent from the legal guardian.
- The person obtaining the consent and the patient or guardian should sign and date the form.
- The signing of the consent form should be witnessed and the witness should sign the form.

The patient has the right to refuse consent and the nurse should ensure that the patient who does so is not coerced into granting consent. Follow your organization's policy regarding steps to take when consent is refused.

If the nurse assesses that after signing the consent the patient is unclear about the procedure or has questions about it, the health care provider who obtained the consent should be contacted and asked to review the procedure with the patient again.

Do Not Resuscitate (DNR) Orders

FAST FACTS in a NUTSHELL

The fact that the family and interdisciplinary team discussed the issue at a team conference and agreed that the patient should not be resuscitated does not substitute for the need for a written order to exist.

A decision not to resuscitate is a medical decision that, like other directives about medical care, requires a physician's order. Because this is a decision about future care, it should be discussed with the competent patient or, in the case of an incompetent patient, the health care proxy. An informal understanding among staff to do a "slow code" if the patient ceases to breathe or a DNR written on the care plan without a supporting medical order is not legal. All staff should be aware of those patients for whom a DNR order exists and adhere to the organization's policy concerning this order.

Invasion of Privacy and Confidentiality

===== *FAST FACTS in a NUTSHELL*

HIPAA contains the first federal privacy standards to protect patients' medical records and other health information provided to health plans, doctors, hospitals, and other health care providers. Developed by the Department of Health and Human Services (HHS), these new standards provide patients with access to their medical records and more control over how their personal health information is used and disclosed. They represent a uniform, federal floor of privacy protections for consumers across the country. HIPAA includes provisions designed to encourage electronic transactions and also requires safeguards to protect the security and confidentiality of health information.

Patients have the right to be free from public view and from having their personal information shared with others. HIPAA has offered a major step in protecting the confidentiality of information. This matter is significant enough that Congress authorized civil and criminal penalties for covered entities that misuse personal health information. States can enact additional privacy protections. When state law requires reporting of infectious diseases and other disclosures, HIPAA does not preempt the state law.

In addition to privacy of medical records, patients should be afforded a reasonable degree of privacy. For nursing home residents, federal regulations describe requirements in regard to residents' privacy, which include their right to:

- Send and receive mail unopened
- Receive visitors
- Use a telephone in private

To protect the patient's privacy:

- Do not allow unauthorized persons to observe or participate in the patient's care without the patient's consent
- Obtain the patient's consent before using photographs or identifying information in a journal article, conference presentation, report, or advertisement

- Take precautions to safeguard the patient's medical record and computer-stored information from unauthorized access
- Do not mention a patient by name or describe in any other identifying manner in social media
- Advise staff members who do not respect patients' privacy or confidentiality of the inappropriateness of their actions
- Knock before entering a closed door of a patient's room

Restraints

A restraint is considered anything that physically or mentally restricts a patient's movement; this could include:

- Protective vests
- Geri-chairs
- Safety bars or belts
- Side rails
- Antipsychotic medications

FAST FACTS in a NUTSHELL

Prior to the 1980s, restraint use was an accepted practice, based on the belief that restraints would prevent falls and injuries. Evidence did not support this belief, and many patients suffered more severe outcomes (e.g., bruises, skin excoriation, asphyxiation) from the use of restraints than they would have if they had fallen or been left to freely wander.

The federal government affected a change in this practice with the Omnibus Budget Reconciliation Act (OBRA), which affected restraint use in nursing homes. Within OBRA was a regulation that stated the nursing home resident *has the right to be free from physical or chemical restraints imposed for the purposes of discipline or convenience and not required to treat the resident's medical condition.*

When patients have behaviors that are at risk of injuring themselves or others, they should be assessed. Their behaviors could arise from a delirium related to pain, an untreated infection, or other medical condition. Addressing the factors that could contribute to the behaviors is essential. If there are no treatable causes identified, alternatives to restraints should be used, such as door alarms to notify staff if the patient wanders off the unit, lowering the bed as much as possible and placing a mat on the floor to buffer a fall, using behavior modification, and providing more frequent staff contact. Consultation with geropsychiatric nurses, psychologists, or psychiatrists could prove beneficial, also.

It must be remembered that improperly used chemical or physical restraints can not only violate regulations concerning their use, but can also result in litigation for false imprisonment and negligence.

OTHER PRACTICE RISKS

Assault and Battery

Every individual has the right to be free from being threatened or touched against his or her will. Assault and battery laws offer people protection in this arena. *Assault* is an intentional threat to cause physical harm by touching a person without his or her consent, whereby the person believes that the threat could be carried out. Telling a patient you are going to refuse to feed him if he doesn't comply with an action and one employee telling another that he will "hurt her" if she tells the supervisor about an incident are examples of assault. *Battery* is the actual act of touching the individual without consent. Performing a diagnostic test without consent and escorting an intoxicated employee from the building by pulling him or her by the arm are forms of battery. Actions that can help to avoid assault and battery include:

- Ensure patients have granted consent for treatments, diagnostic tests, and other care measures that exceed basic, routine care
- Respect patients' right to refuse care
- Ensure caregivers do not make threats to convince patients to comply with care or change their behaviors
- Do not touch employees or visitors without their approval.

Defamation

Communicating, verbally or in writing, a message that injures a person's reputation, is considered defamation. *Libel* is the written form of defamation and *slander* the verbal form.

Making a true statement about someone to a third party who has legitimate reason to receive the information is not considered defamation. For example, if an employer is asked on a reference about a nurse's work habits, it is fine to state that a nurse was terminated for making eight medication errors in one month. However, if the employer suspected that the nurse stole narcotics but this was never proven, to write on the reference that the nurse "cannot be trusted with narcotics" or that the nurse "was believed to have stolen narcotics" could be considered libel.

FAST FACTS in a NUTSHELL

Social media offers new venues in which defamation can occur. Posting or sending critical and injurious comments about a coworker, patient, or patient's family member can lead to claims of defamation. Nurses need to be cautious of this and advise other staff members to avoid this behavior.

To reduce the risk for defamation, avoid:

- Making untrue or negative comments about coworkers, patients, and visitors
- Writing criticisms or judgments about other staff in patients' records
- Giving a reference on an employee without having evidence that the employee has granted consent for this
- Stating items that are untrue or unproven on references

False Imprisonment

Detaining or restraining a person without good cause is considered false imprisonment. This can occur if a competent patient wishes to leave the hospital but the staff block the patient from leaving the room because they are concerned that he or she will not receive the necessary medications. It also can involve employees, as can happen if an employee is suspected of theft and other employees lock him or her in a room until the police arrive. There are special provisions for health care facilities to detain a patient, such as if the patient has a contagious disease or has a mental illness that makes him or her at risk of harming self or others.

FAST FACTS in a NUTSHELL

When a competent patient decides to leave a health care facility against medical advice, this information should be documented in the patient's record. It may be wise to notify the patient's next of kin or responsible party so that he or she may intervene and assist the person.

Incidents/Accidents

An *incident* is anything that happens out of the ordinary, such as the loss of personal property, improper administration of a medication, resident or employee slip on the floor, and a patient wandering away from the facility. An *accident* implies that an unintentional injury has resulted; for example, the patient who was given an improper medication develops a reaction, the person who slipped on the floor has a gash on the head, and the patient who wandered off the premises becomes hypothermic.

All incidents and accidents must be documented on the form designated by the facility. No matter how minor or insignificant incidents and accidents seem, they should be documented. The accuracy and appropriateness of the incident and accident documentation can prove invaluable to the facility should litigation result.

FAST FACTS in a NUTSHELL

When completing an incident/accident form, it is important to document facts and observations without making conclusions.

[Clinical Snapshot]

Nurse A goes into a patient's room and finds the patient on the floor. As Nurse A didn't witness the incident, she needs to state what she observed. If the patient or witnesses offer explanations of what occurred, Nurse A should document the statements as quotations and attribute the comments to the persons making the statements. Her proper documentation of the incident will read, "Patient found lying on floor along side of bed. Patient states, 'I slipped out of bed when I tried to stand.'"

The nursing management and quality assurance staff should review incident and accident reports to identify problems and trends. Monthly tabulation of incidents and accidents by unit can aid in identifying patient changes and problem areas; for instance, a rise in employee back injuries over the past 3 months could indicate the need for inservice education on the topic of body mechanics, or it could reflect a change toward a more obese patient population. By investigating trends identified on incident and accident reports the nursing department can keep abreast of relevant practice issues.

Malpractice/Negligence

Nurses are responsible for ensuring their practice is consistent with good standards of care. Standards of care are based on current best practices, available through sources such as journal articles and professional associations (e.g., standards developed and published by the Joint Commission, American Nurses Association, and American Association for Long Term Care Nursing).

Malpractice can be claimed if there is a deviation from a standard of care that results in harm to a patient. It can arise from commission, in which a procedure is performed inappropriately, or omission whereby a procedure that should have been performed was not. The fact that a procedure was performed inappropriately in itself is not grounds for malpractice. For malpractice to occur there must be:

- *Duty:* A relationship that exists between the patient and nurse whereby the patient has contracted for/agreed to the services and the nurse is responsible to perform those services.
- *Negligence:* The action fails to meet the acceptable standard for that action.
- *Injury:* Harm occurs as a result of the negligent action.

FAST FACTS in a NUTSHELL

In malpractice cases, harm can include physical or mental harm to the patient, or a violation of the patient's rights.

To reduce the risk of malpractice the nurse should:

- Know and adhere to the approved policies and procedures of the employing agency and the standards expressed in regulations pertaining to the practice setting
- Know and adhere to the standards of practice expressed in the state's nurse practice act
- Avoid performing tasks that exceed licensure, knowledge, skills, and available resources
- Review the plan of care before giving care
- Identify the patient before providing care
- Follow medical orders as written; consult with the medical provider if an order is unclear or inappropriate
- Monitor patients' status; promptly identify, assess, and report changes in status
- Keep patients informed and give them explanations of care activities
- Document accurately and thoroughly
- Maintain competency by keeping current on nursing practice
- Delegate carefully based on known capabilities of staff; follow up on delegated tasks

FAST FACTS in a NUTSHELL

It is useful for nurses to carry their own malpractice insurance, as there may be conditions in which the employer's insurance will not provide coverage, the nurse could offer services outside the formal work setting, and a jury could award damages that exceed the limits of the employer's policy, thereby leaving the nurse liable for the balance.

Respondeat Superior (Supervision)

Respondeat superior comes from the Latin term meaning "let the superior reply," and describes the legal relationship between an employer and employee.

FAST FACTS in a NUTSHELL

An employer will be liable for acts an employee committed while within the scope of employment. The liability of an employer for the acts of an employee is called vicarious liability.

In many geriatric care settings, nurses are responsible for many unlicensed personnel and can be liable for the wrongful actions of an employee if the nurse who has responsibility for supervising or delegating to an employee:

- Assigns a task to the employee that the employee is not licensed or competent to perform
- Fails to ensure that a delegated task was properly completed
- Allows the employee to engage in an improper or illegal activity without intervening

This does not imply that the supervisor or organization is responsible for all wrongful acts of employees under their supervision. For example, a nursing assistant in a nursing home may have been trained to insert a nasogastric tube while a medical corpsman; however, this task is not within the scope of practice or job description of nursing assistants in the facility. If, without the supervisor's knowledge, the nursing assistant proceeds to reinsert a nasogastric tube independently, the supervisor and employer may not be found liable.

Nurses need to be aware of the competencies and scope of practice for employees for whom they are responsible. They also need to ensure that they have adequate resources to allow them and the employees they supervise to perform their jobs safely and properly.

Telephone Orders

Many care settings do not have physicians on the premises 24 hours each day, thus, nursing staff must rely on telephone communication to inform physicians of changes in the patient's status and to receive instructions from physicians. Accepting telephone orders can pose risks for nurses in that the order can be heard incorrectly, given incorrectly, or the physician could later deny the order was given.

It is wise for facilities and agencies to have policies concerning who may accept telephone orders and the conditions accompanying the order.

Some recommendations that can aid in reducing the risks associated with telephone orders are:

- Follow the employer's policies concerning who may accept telephone orders and the conditions accompanying the order.
- Designate certain staff or levels of staff who may telephone physicians and accept telephone orders.
- Assess the patient prior to the telephone communication and have the assessment data readily available during the conversation.
- Inform the physician of the patient's current status, vital signs, and significant observations.
- Remind the physician of the medications currently being administered to the patient.
- Speak directly to the physician, not through office staff.
- Write the order as it is being given and read it back to the physician.

- Consider having the physician fax the order, to have a written record and ensure accuracy of the communication.
- Question orders that seem unsafe or inappropriate. If the physician demands that the order be followed despite your objection, inform the physician that you will not implement the order until you can verify it with the medical director or another physician.
- Write the entire order on the order sheet, identifying it as a telephone order. Sign your name.
- Remind the physician to sign the order within 24 hours.

FAST FACTS in a NUTSHELL

If a recording of the telephone order is to be made, one of two conditions must be met to allow this recording to be admissible in court in the event of litigation:

- *The person must be informed that the call is being recorded and will be saved in the event of litigation.*
- *Special recording equipment must be used that sounds a tone to indicate to the parties on the telephone line that the call is being recorded.*

18

End of Life Care

When caring for people of advanced age, particularly those with health conditions, nurses are certain to encounter patients who are near the end of their lives. In a health care system in which medical knowledge and technology have enabled people to live to advanced ages and be kept alive in serious states, death sometimes can be viewed as a problem to be overcome rather than a natural part of life's trajectory. Yet, there comes a time when aggressive treatment is merely prolonging the time when death occurs rather than extending a life of quality. At this time, the focus shifts to end of life care in which the older individual is supported through the dying process with peace, comfort, and dignity. Regardless of the setting in which they work, nurses play a significant role in providing palliative care that helps older people and their loved ones navigate through this significant life event.

Objectives

In this chapter you will learn to:

1. Describe the purpose of advance directives
2. List considerations in conducting a pain assessment
3. Describe signs of pain in persons with dementia
4. List nonpharmacologic measures that can be used to reduce pain
5. Describe nursing measures to relieve dyspnea, poor intake, constipation, and fatigue
6. List useful interventions for each of Elisabeth Kübler-Ross' stages of dying
7. Describe cultural and religious practices related to death and dying
8. Discuss support that the family may need
9. List signs of imminent death

DISCUSSING END OF LIFE ISSUES

Ideally, individuals discuss their preferences about end of life care with their families and health care providers prior to the time it is needed; however, discussions about death and dying are often difficult for people. When such discussions have been neglected, older adults risk receiving care that they would not have desired and their loved ones are faced with the burden of having to make decisions at a time of crisis. Nurses can play an important role in facilitating end of life discussions and ensuring individuals' desires are understood.

FAST FACTS in a NUTSHELL

When the older adult has not developed an advance directive and discussed end of life care preferences with family members the nurse can introduce these topics.

[Clinical Snapshot]

Mr. E acknowledged upon admission to the hospital that he had no advance directive, as he did not think he needed one. Having heard Mr. E discuss his desire to not burden his family, the nurse discussed the usefulness of the advance directive in ensuring Mr. E's desires were known and sparing his family the headaches of making decisions without an understanding of his wishes. By assessing Mr. E's readiness to discuss the issue and relating it to something important to him, the nurse was able to engage Mr. E in a meaningful discussion.

Advance directives are legally binding documents in which competent people state the medical care and interventions they would or would not want to receive in the event they are unable to competently make or state their preferences. As part of the advance directive, people can develop a *durable power of attorney* in which they designate a person to make decisions on their behalf should they be incapable of making their own decisions in the form of a health care proxy (also referred to as a proxy decision maker).

The Patient Self-Determination Act, enacted by Congress in 1990 and becoming effective in 1991, required that health care organizations had to:

- Inform patients of their right to make health care decisions and refuse treatments
- Ask patients if they had completed an advance directive
- Provide written information about their state's provisions for implementing advance directives
- Include documentation of patients' advance directives in their medical records
- Educate the staff and community about advance directives

The nurse plays an important role in inquiring about this document and facilitating discussions with patients about their desires. If the nurse identifies that the patient is uncomfortable with what has been expressed in the advance directive or wishes to change it, the patient should be assisted in doing so. A copy of the patient's advance directive should be included in the medical record and all members of the interdisciplinary team should be aware of and respect its contents.

=========================== *FAST FACTS in a NUTSHELL*

A do not resuscitate (DNR) order is a medical order that directs health care providers to not perform cardiopulmonary resuscitation if the patient ceases to have a heartbeat and respirations. It does not prevent providers from delivering treatment to the patient if the patient is still alive.

PAIN MANAGEMENT

A primary concern of the person who is dying and his or her loved ones is the management of pain. Pain can weaken the patient's ability to not only perform basic physical functions of life, but also to engage in important emotional, psychological, and spiritual activities. Unrelieved pain can increase fatigue, stress, and depression, and reduce the person's ability to make decisions and exercise control.

Pain can be *nociceptive* or *neuropathic*. Nociceptive involves stimulation of pain receptors (e.g., organs, bones, muscles) and can be:

- *Visceral:* this is related to organs and often is described as deep, a dull ache, or squeezing
- *Somatic:* results from stimuli in skin, muscles, and bones; is well localized; described as sharp or aching

Neuropathic pain is related to the nervous system (e.g., diabetic neuropathy, sciatica, phantom limb) and is described as burning, tingling, or shooting.

Pain assessment is crucial and must be performed regularly. Considerations related to pain assessment include:

- The patient's level of pain can dramatically change in a relatively short time frame.
- Cultural background, diagnosis, emotional state, cognitive function, spiritual beliefs, and experience with illness are

among the factors that can influence a patient's perception and expression of pain.

- In addition to verbalizations of pain or discomfort, nonverbal signs of pain can include delirium, nausea, irritability, sleep disturbances, reduced activity, diaphoresis, pallor, poor appetite, grimacing, withdrawal, restlessness, and anxiety.
- Pain is considered to be present if the patient says it is.

A variety of scales can be used to aid in assessing pain. Basically, asking the patient to rate the pain on a scale of 0 to 10, with 0 being no pain and 10 being the most severe, can aid in assessing pain severity. Using the same rating scale consistently aids in providing a more reliable basis for comparison.

Patients with dementia may be unable to describe their pain, so nurses need to observe for signs that indicate pain; these could include:

- Resisting care
- Clenched fists
- Facial grimacing
- Hitting, kicking, biting, pushing
- Uncontrollable behaviors
- Rigidity
- Moaning
- Crying, yelling
- Hyperventilation
- Labored respirations

Detailed descriptions of observations should be noted, as well as measures that alleviated the symptoms.

Pain management for patients at the end of their lives should focus on preventing pain. This can be achieved by documenting the time period after which the analgesic is administered when pain returns, and developing a schedule that provides the analgesic prior to the anticipated time of the onset of pain. This preventive approach to pain management not only facilitates comfort and saves energy, but could reduce the amount of analgesics that are needed.

The analgesic prescribed will depend on the intensity of pain and the risk of adverse effects. Aspirin or acetaminophen can be used to relieve mild pain, codeine or oxycodone can be used for moderate pain, and morphine or hydromorphone may be prescribed for severe pain. Due to their high incidence of adverse reactions, meperidine and pentazocine are contraindicated for pain control in older adults.

Nonpharmacologic measures can be beneficial in relieving pain or reducing the amount of analgesic used. Box 18.1 describes some of the measures that could be used.

Box 18.1 Nonpharmacologic Therapies to Relieve Pain

Acupressure: a traditional Chinese medicine bodywork technique based on the same principles as acupuncture. It involves placing physical pressure on different pressure points on the body to unblock energy pathways (meridian). The theory is that disease or illness results from the blockage or obstructions of the pathways. Therefore, clearing the blockages allows the chi to run freely through the meridians and restores health.

Acupuncture: a traditional Chinese medicine technique that inserts pins to unblock the pathways (meridians or channels) at specific juncture points through which the chi or life force flows. It has been determined that acupuncture stimulates physical responses, such as changing brain activity, blood chemistry, endocrine functions, blood pressure, heart rate, and immune system response. It can offer pain relief by triggering endorphin production.

Biofeedback: a process of learned control of physical responses of the body. Through the use of instruments a person is trained to relax and monitor changes through certain feedback devices. Meditation, relaxation, and visualization techniques are taught, and these techniques ultimately teach psychological control over physical processes.

Guided imagery: based on the belief that images can be created in the mind that can influence the body to relieve symptoms and promote relaxation. A person can use guided imagery alone or be led by a practitioner.

(continued)

Massage: the therapeutic practice of kneading or manipulating soft tissue and muscles with the intent of increasing health and well-being and assisting the body in healing. It is understood that besides stretching and loosening muscle and connective tissue, the action of massage also improves blood flow and the flow of lymph throughout the body, speeds the metabolism of waste products, promotes the circulation of oxygen and nutrients to cells and tissues, and stimulates the release of endorphins and serotonin in the brain and nervous system.

Meditation: focused attention of the mind to help the body reach a relaxed state. The person may deep breathe and repeat a particular word or phrase.

Reiki: a form of healing in which the Reiki master channels energy to another individual.

Therapeutic touch (healing touch): based on the principle that people are energy fields who can transfer energy to one another to promote healing. The practitioner's hands do not directly touch the patient, but are held several inches above the body surface within the energy field and positioned in purposeful ways. A core element of therapeutic touch is the mindset or intent of the practitioner to help.

FAST FACTS in a NUTSHELL

For the dying individual, a balance should be sought between sufficient pain relief to prevent suffering and enabling the person sufficient alertness to interact with loved ones and exercise a level of control that he or she desires.

PHYSICAL SYMPTOMS AND THEIR MANAGEMENT

Dyspnea

Basic physical functions can be affected by the dying process, one of which is respiration. Pleural effusion, deteriorating blood gases, and the effects of disease processes can cause respiratory distress. In addition to the physical discomfort this produces, the anxiety and feelings of helplessness produced by the inability to adequately breathe leads to psychological distress. Relief can be obtained by:

- Elevating the head of the bed
- Scheduling activities to allow rest between activities
- Guiding the patient in relaxation exercises
- Administering oxygen as ordered
- Administering medications as ordered (atropine or furosemide may be administered to reduce bronchial secretions; narcotics may be used for their ability to control respiratory symptoms by blunting the medullary response)

_____ *FAST FACTS in a NUTSHELL*

A rattling sound, often referred to as a death rattle, can occur in the days or hours preceding death. This occurs due to saliva pooling in the back of the throat and the patient being too weak to expel the secretions. Although this can be distressing for others, it is not believed to be painful for the patient.

Poor Intake

Anorexia, nausea, vomiting, and weakness contribute to poor nutritional intake. Assistance with feeding may be beneficial, as may providing frequent, smaller-portioned meals rather than three large ones. Nausea and vomiting can be controlled with the use of antiemetics and antihistamines; ginger may be effective as a natural antiemetic. Special food items that the person enjoys should be offered and the environment should be controlled to provide pleasant, odor-free surroundings. If pain is restricting food intake, the use of analgesics could prove useful. Frequent oral hygiene can provide comfort. The person should be encouraged but not forced to eat. Forced feeding could increase discomfort and cause aspiration of food.

Ceasing to ingest food and fluids often occurs in the days prior to death. Some people may make a conscious decision to stop eating as a means to hasten death.

=========================== *FAST FACTS in a NUTSHELL*

> *Family members and caregivers should be reassured that the dying patient's lack of eating and drinking does not mean the patient will experience more discomfort. Ketosis occurs when there has been extended lack of intake, which depresses hunger sensations and causes euphoria in some people. Dehydration can reduce secretions, thereby easing respirations, and may release endorphins.*

Constipation

Low intake, dehydration, immobility, medications, and the effects of disease processes can cause constipation. This can contribute to additional discomfort for the patient. The patient should be regularly assessed for constipation; signs include:

- Reduced frequency of bowel movements
- Straining to pass a stool
- Abdominal discomfort
- Abdominal fullness
- Reduced bowel sounds
- Presence of an impaction

Being a common occurrence near the end of life, efforts to promote bowel elimination should be incorporated into the care plan.

Fatigue

The lack of physical strength and endurance are among the most common symptoms at the end of life. Assess for and address other factors that could contribute to fatigue, such as dehydration, hypoxia, poor sleep patterns, fever, anxiety, and medication side effects. Schedule care activities to afford rest between activities.

EMOTIONAL SUPPORT

More than four decades ago, Elisabeth Kübler-Ross identified five stages that dying individuals experience as coping mechanisms (Kübler-Ross, 1969). Because the dying experience is unique for each person, not everyone will progress through these stages similarly or in sequence; however, knowing these stages can assist in understanding reactions patients demonstrate and guide supportive actions by the nurse. The stages are:

Denial: The reality that the end of life is near can be too overwhelming for people to accept. As a means to cope with their feelings and mobilize their defenses they may deny this reality. Not only can this occur upon first learning of a diagnosis, but also at various times during the course of the illness as emotional strength fluctuates. It is important for the nurse to be patient and allow patients to process their feelings and to be available for support.

Anger: Realizing the limited amount of life that remains, patients may become angry about their situation. This anger often is displaced to those the patients are most comfortable with, such as family members and regular caregivers. Nursing staff needs to remember and help families understand that it is the situation, not them, that is the root cause of the anger. Allowing patients to express their feelings without offering judgment, anticipating needs, and maintaining regular contact are important actions during this stage.

Bargaining: During this stage patients may resort to negotiating for more time by committing to certain actions. For example, they may agree to attend church more regularly if God will allow them to live through one more Christmas, or donate money to a charity if their cancer can go into remission. Patients may need to be protected from being taken advantage of by unscrupulous people who may offer dangerous options or false hope for their own financial gain.

Depression: Particularly for older adults who often are experiencing many losses in their lives as a result of age-related factors, depression can develop as they experience the reality of death, uncomfortable symptoms, and declining status. Usually this is a silent depression, not aided by cheerful comments. Family and friends of dying patients who are in this stage need to understand that comments like, "Come on now, cheer up," or "You should look at the light side," are not helpful. Rather, spending time with patients, even sitting in silence with them, can be beneficial. Because they may feel helpless and uncomfortable, family and friends may need extra support when patients are in this stage.

Acceptance: This stage implies that patients have come to terms with the reality of their situation and are not fighting it. This does not imply that they are happy with the situation, but rather, than they have achieved a sense of peace with it.

Family and friends need to understand these stages and be assisted with identifying helpful actions that can assist at various stages. Describing these emotional responses as therapeutic steps to adjusting to the loss of life can aid them in accepting patients' behaviors.

FAST FACTS in a NUTSHELL

Hope can permeate every stage of the dying process. It can involve individuals feeling confident that they will be well taken care of as they are dying, trusting that their children will take care of their spouses after they are gone, or believing that they will be facing eternal life in heaven.

Patients should be encouraged and aided to express their feelings. This can be done by asking questions (e.g., "What types of things concern you right now?" "How do you feel about what the doctor just told you?") and being available to listen. Listening is facilitated by:

• Sitting on eye level with the patient
• Intentionally focusing attention on the patient

- Allocating uninterrupted time to invest with the patient
- Allowing the patient to express feelings without interrupting
- Not making assumptions about what the patient is going to say
- Fully hearing what the patient is saying before thinking about a response

Holding hands, stroking a cheek, gently massaging a shoulder, and other acts of physical touch can convey caring and facilitate patients' expression of feelings.

SPIRITUAL SUPPORT

FAST FACTS in a NUTSHELL

Spirituality is not the same as religion. Religion involves a set of beliefs that is expressed through doctrine, rites, and rituals. Spirituality involves finding meaning in something beyond oneself; it may not be associated with belief in a deity or specific faith.

As death nears, people may have as much concern for their spiritual needs as their physical care. This can involve issues such as making peace with God, understanding the meaning that their lives have had, and resolving conflicts with friends and family. Both dying patients and their loved ones may have the need to express their feelings toward each other and describe the importance they have had in each others' lives. Many patients will appreciate visits from their clergy and members of their faith communities.

Various religions and cultures have specific practices related to death and dying (see Boxes 18.2 and 18.3). Nurses should honor these, recognizing that not all members of a specific religious or cultural group will adhere to all the practices customary for the group and avoid stereotypes.

Box 18.2   Religious Practices at the End of Life

Religious Affiliation	Beliefs and Practices Related to Death
Baptist	Prayer, communion
Buddhist	Last rites by Buddhist priest; forgiveness encouraged to aid in dying with peace; after death leave body alone as long as possible to avoid disturbing consciousness during transition from death to new life
Catholic	Prayer, last rites by priest
Christian Scientist	Visit from Christian Science reader
Episcopal	Prayer, communion, confession, last rites
Friends (Quakers)	Individual communicates with God directly, no belief in afterlife
Hindu	Visit by priest to perform ritual of tying thread around neck or wrist, water put in mouth, family cleanses body after death, cremation accepted
Judaism	After death, body washed by Orthodox Jew, someone stays with body until it is buried, cremation not allowed
Lutheran	Prayer, last rites
Mormon	Baptism and preaching to deceased
Orthodox (Greek, Russian)	Prayer, communion, last rites (Holy Unction) by priest; cremation not allowed
Pentecostal	Prayer, communion
Presbyterian	Prayer, last rites

Box 18.3   Cultural Practices at the End of Life

Cultural Group	Beliefs and Practices Related to Death
African American	Emotional displays (e.g., collapsing, screaming) in reaction to death
Cubans, Filipinos, Mexicans	Large group of relatives and friends are with dying person, place religious artifacts around person, light candles as a means of guiding spirit to afterlife; may have strong emotional and hyperkinetic reaction to learning of death of loved one
Haitians	Attempt for all family to gather at bedside and pray; family members may cry uncontrollably
Indians, Hindus	Death rites performed by priest assisted by eldest son and other male relatives; women may display loud wailing
Japanese	Family members gather at time of death and stay at bedside; eldest son directs activities
Koreans	Family members gather at time of death, stay at bedside, and assist with care
Navajo Indians	Do not talk directly about the person dying but discuss the issue in the third person, as talking about death to the person implies that one wishes the person to die
Puerto Ricans	Head of family receives notice of death and communicates to others; family may want to stay with and touch body before it is removed
Vietnamese	Do not want flowers in room of the dying person, as they are considered part of the rites of the dead

SUPPORTING FAMILY

Today's families have fewer direct experiences with death than previous generations due to nuclear family structures, mobility of family members, and improved management of health conditions that has reduced mortality rates. In addition, most deaths occur in a hospital or nursing home setting, thereby reducing the intimate experience that family members have with the dying process of loved ones.

Communication is of significant importance to the family. Unless there is objection by the patient, the family needs to be informed about the patient's status. Family conferences provide an opportunity to discuss changes in condition, care needs, and goals. Family members should be encouraged to discuss their feelings and needs.

Family members who serve the role of caregiver need information and education to understand:

- The disease and its effects
- Symptoms and their meaning
- Treatments and medications (e.g., purpose, how they are administered, side effects, precautions)
- Caregiving skills (e.g., positioning, lifting, bathing tips)
- How to meet nutritional needs
- Anticipated physical and emotional reactions
- The need for their own self-care

Family caregivers also need to understand their need for respite and assistance in finding resources to provide help.

_____ *FAST FACTS in a NUTSHELL*

Sometimes one sibling may absorb more responsibility for caregiving of a parent than other siblings, but be reluctant to ask for assistance. The nurse may suggest a family meeting in which the nurse leads the discussion, introduces the topic of shared responsibilities, and guides the development of a plan in which all family members commit to some role.

After the death, the family may need support during their bereavement period. Encourage the open expression of feelings. Referrals to clergy, grief support groups, and organizations that could assist with financial and other types of assistance could prove beneficial.

DEATH

Within days of imminent death, the patient will display signs of active dying, which include:

- Altered breathing pattern, such as dyspnea, shallow respirations, Cheyne-Stokes respirations, gurgling or rattling sounds with breathing
- Reduced responsiveness and level of consciousness
- Confusion, hallucinations
- Weak, irregular pulse
- Reduced blood pressure
- Disinterest in and reluctance to consume food and fluid
- Bladder and bowel incontinence, anuria
- Distorted vision, slow or no pupil response to light
- Diminished reflexes
- Cold extremities
- Skin pallor and mottling
- Profuse perspiration

When death occurs there will be an absence of heartbeat and respirations, eyes may be open with dilated pupils, the mouth may drop open, and there will be no response to stimuli. Follow your organization's procedure for the process of legal pronouncement of death and release of the body to the mortuary.

Family should be provided ample time to be with the deceased person. It is helpful to remove visible tubing and medical devices and apply a clean sheet to cover the body prior to having the family enter to say their farewells. The body should be prepared in the manner preferred based on cultural and spiritual preferences. The eyes should be gently closed and the head slightly elevated to reduce discoloration. Dentures should be placed in the mouth if they have been removed and the mouth closed; placing a rolled towel under the chin can assist with keeping the mouth closed. Maintain the patient's body in a supine position.

Documentation should include time of death, the physician who pronounced the patient dead, and any other significant information. The patient's personal belongings should be given to the family and documentation should list what was given and who accepted the patient's items.

FAST FACTS in a NUTSHELL

Staff who have cared for a patient for long time often are impacted by the patient's death and will need time to grieve and opportunities to express their feelings. Likewise, in a nursing home or assisted living community in which residents have lived together for a period of time, they also will be impacted by the death. Memorial services within the facility and posting a table in the lobby in which the deceased person's photograph, obituary, and a book in which sympathies can be expressed can aid in helping others to say their farewells and honor the deceased person.

19

Geriatric Nursing in Various Care Settings

Older adults receive services in virtually all clinical settings and their increasing numbers will challenge growing numbers of nurses to be engaged in geriatric care in the future. In addition, there has been a growth of geriatric-specific services along the continuum of care that has created new roles for geriatric nurses. Regardless of the clinical setting, it is important when considering service delivery to older adults that:

- *Care be based on the latest evidence-based geriatric practice*
- *Comprehensive assessments be done to provide holistic individualized care*
- *Patients be informed about and engaged in their care to the fullest extent possible*
- *Privacy and the rights of the patient as an adult be respected*
- *Care be adjusted to accommodate age-related changes; health status; level of independent function; patient preferences; and cultural, religious, educational, and ethnic backgrounds.*

Today's older adults are better informed and have greater expectations of health care providers than previous generations. They not only desire to have conditions treated, but want to be equipped with knowledge and competencies to engage in health practices based on the most current evidence. Nurses are the ideal professionals to meet these demands and ensure that care addresses holistic needs.

Objectives

In this chapter you will learn to:

1. Identify the continuum of services available to older adults
2. List specific risks for older hospitalized patients
3. Describe considerations to promote the safety and comfort of older hospitalized patients
4. Describe factors to consider in discharge planning
5. List regulatory requirements for nursing homes described in Omnibus Budget Reconciliation Act (OBRA)
6. Describe measures that can assist the nursing home admission process for residents and their families
7. Identify basic principles and practices of nursing home culture change
8. List the types of services provided in assisted living communities
9. List potential problems that could be identified by home health nurses

HOSPITAL CARE

FAST FACTS in a NUTSHELL

As compared to other age groups, persons over the age of 65 years have a higher rate of hospitalization and longer lengths of stay (Centers for Disease Control and Prevention, 2013a).

Advanced age causes people to have a greater likelihood of developing system malfunctions and diseases that require hospitalizations for diagnostic and treatment purposes. Older patients are likely to have chronic conditions and disabilities that can affect the course of their hospitalization and increase their risk for complications such as nosocomial infections, adverse drug events, and cognitive decline (Wilson et al., 2012). These complications are often associated with poorer outcomes after discharge. In addition, the increased time required to recover from acute episodes, combined with comorbidities, can prevent older patients from returning home and cause them to require post-hospital institutional care. The following are risks of particular concern in caring for the older hospitalized patient.

Delirium

Older adults could have altered cognition upon arrival to the hospital as a result of the acute episode. This must be differentiated from dementia; if hospital staff assume that altered cognition is normal for older adults or that the patient has a dementia, they may not realize that a potentially reversible problem is present that warrants treatment and fail to identify underlying conditions.

Delirium can also occur during a hospitalization due to fluid and electrolyte disturbances, polypharmacy, adverse drug reactions, infections, stress, the use of restraints, and a variety of other causes (see Chapter 11). It is important to obtain a history of what the patient's mental status typically was prior to admission and at admission so that changes can be identified. Older patients tend to develop delirium as a postoperative complication more than younger age groups.

Monitoring the patient's status and identifying changes promptly can assist in preventing delirium. As older adults may react to medications (particularly sedatives and psychotropics) by developing a delirium, alternatives to medications should be used whenever possible.

FAST FACTS in a NUTSHELL

Chemically or physically restraining an older person could cause a delirium. When a patient has behaviors that are difficult to control, alternative measures to calm the patient should be attempted. These could include explaining caregiving activities before implementing them, offering a massage, providing comfort measures, or having a family or staff member stay with the patient to supervise his behavior and offer calming reassurance.

Falls

A variety of factors could contribute to patients falling in the hospital. These could include:

- Unfamiliar environment
- Dizziness
- Weakness
- Orthosatic hypotension
- Delirium
- Restraints (e.g., bedrails, psychotropic medications)
- Pain
- Sedation
- Lack of assistance with toileting, transfers

Patients should be regularly assessed for fall risk and plans developed to address identified risks.

=========================== *FAST FACTS in a NUTSHELL*

Falls resulting in hip fractures are a particular risk to patients over age 85.

Close supervision and providing necessary assistance are useful measures in reducing the risk for falls. Encouraging activity and exercise can aid in preventing the loss of strength and mobility. Assistive devices that the patient needs to use should be readily available. Providing proper footwear and encouraging patients to use handrails can also prove beneficial.

=========================== *FAST FACTS in a NUTSHELL*

Unless contraindicated, a patient who has used a walker prior to hospital admission should have the walker available for use during the hospitalization. Having the patient use a wheelchair rather than walker for the purpose of convenience or speed of transit could cause an unnecessary loss of strength and mobility. Consulting with physical therapy could assist in determining the appropriateness of using various mobility aids.

Pressure Ulcers

Changes to the integumentary system contribute to a high risk for pressure ulcers in most older adults; bedrest, restricted mobility, sedation, incontinence, diaphoresis, and inadequate attention to turning and repositioning are among the factors that heighten this risk during hospitalization.

FAST FACTS in a NUTSHELL

During acute hospitalizations there are many serious monitoring and treatment activities that are done. It is easy for a basic nursing measure such as repositioning to be overlooked among these critical activities. In addition, IV, catheter, and oxygen tubing, along with dressings and casts, could make changes in position difficult. Despite these challenges, older patients need turning and repositioning frequently.

Long surgeries in which the older patient is in the same position on a hard operating room table for an extended period of time can initiate pressure ulcer development. Padding the patient's bony prominences can aid in preventing pressure ulcers and bone discomfort postoperatively. Basic pressure ulcer prevention measures should be heeded throughout the hospitalization (see Chapter 9).

Infection

Older adults are at high risk for hospital-acquired infections. Strict adherence to infection control measures is vital. Hospital staff should be aware that infections could present differently in the older patient. For example, fever may not be evident due to lower normal body temperatures, respiratory signs (e.g., productive cough, chest pain) may not accompany pneumonia, and the severity of pain reported may not correlate with the degree of inflammation. Delirium may be the primary sign that an infection exists, and if the patient's norm isn't known, this could be missed and diagnosis delayed.

FAST FACTS in a NUTSHELL

Strengthening the older patient's nutritional status, ensuring no untreated infection is present, and teaching measures that can be used postoperatively (e.g., deep breathing, repositioning techniques) are beneficial preoperative actions to reduce the risk of infection postoperatively.

Dehydration

Many older adults have reduced thirst sensations, which can affect their ability to consume sufficient fluids under any condition. When hospitalized or experiencing an acute illness, the risk of dehydration becomes greater due to nausea, vomiting, NPO status, pain, diuresis, or inability to independently reach and consume fluids. Close monitoring of intake and output should be routine nursing actions for older patients.

Reduced Level of Independence

Illnesses and injuries can reduce the functional capacity of older adults. This can be compounded by caregiver expectations that patients are unable to engage in self-care activities, or that patients may risk injuries by engaging in self-care activities, and staff performing tasks that patients could perform independently in an effort to save time or due to stereotypes about older persons. Even brief periods of reduced engagement in the activities of daily living can result in long-term declines in functional capacity. Regardless of how basic the task, such as walking to the bathroom rather than using a bedpan or feeding oneself, patients should be encouraged to perform as many activities independently as possible.

It is beneficial to involve physical and occupational therapists in the care of older patients. They can devise appropriate exercise plans and identify assistive devices that can foster independent function. Early mobilization and participation in self-care activities can enhance a faster return to independent function and affect patients' discharge.

Constipation

Many older individuals have challenges with constipation in the absence of illness. During acute illness and hospitalization the risk of constipation rises due to reduced activity, dietary modifications, the effects of medications, and the inability to use or reach a commode. Monitoring of elimination should be a routine measure. It is useful to promote the intake of food items that could enhance bowel elimination; if this is not possible, a laxative may be necessary. Extended periods of constipation are not only uncomfortable for patients, but could risk fecal impaction.

========= *FAST FACTS in a NUTSHELL*

With a fecal impaction, the oozing of liquids around the impaction could be mistaken for diarrhea. If antidiarrheal medications are given to address this symptom, the patient's problem is compounded, and complications, such as an intestinal blockage, could result. This emphasizes the importance of monitoring bowel elimination and performing a good physical assessment before determining the patient's problem.

Incontinence

There is a risk for functional incontinence when an older adult is hospitalized due to inaccessible toilet facilities, lack of assistance, immobility, sedation, diuresis, or altered cognition. It should not be assumed that this is a normal or permanent condition for older patients. As most older adults require frequent urination under normal conditions, toileting assistance should be anticipated approximately every 2 hours during the day and at least once during the night. When incontinence develops during a hospitalization, its cause should be evaluated and corrected as soon as possible.

Special Risks for Older Patients Undergoing Surgery

Close monitoring during surgery is especially important, as anesthesia depresses the functions of the cardiovascular and respiratory systems that already work less efficiently due to age-related changes. Inhaled anesthesia agents tend to remain in older patients for a longer period of time; therefore, turning and deep breathing as soon as possible postoperatively can assist in eliminating these agents and enhancing recovery.

The lower body temperatures, reduced adipose tissue to provide natural insulation, medications that depress function, and cool temperatures of operating rooms can heighten the risk for hypothermia. These factors and the shivering that could occur can increase the demands on the heart and lungs and reduce oxygen circulation. Hypothermic states also delay awakening from anesthesia and return of reflexes. Monitoring patients' temperatures during and following surgery and keeping the body warm can be beneficial.

FAST FACTS in a NUTSHELL

Warming the body during the intraoperative and early postoperative periods has been shown to raise core temperatures and reduce the incidence of hypothermia (Horn et al., 2012; Yang et al., 2012).

As older adults have a reduced ability to manage physiologic stress, symptoms of shock and hemorrhage need to be observed for and promptly addressed. Older adults may display hypoxia through restlessness; it is important that this restlessness not be interpreted as pain and a narcotic administered, as this could depress respirations and oxygen supply to a greater extent. Many older patients benefit from the administration of low levels of oxygen postoperatively.

Postoperative complications that older patients are at particular risk for developing and that must be observed for include:

- Delirium
- Pneumonia
- Pulmonary emboli
- Atelectasis
- Embolus, thrombus
- Myocardial infarction
- Arrhythmias
- Pressure ulcers

- Drug-induced renal failure (associated with cimetidine, digoxin, aminoglycosides, cephalosporins, ampicillin, neuromuscular-blocking agents)
- Paralytic ileus (signs include fever, dehydration, abdominal tenderness, and distension)

Discharge Planning

Discharge planning is a consideration upon admission. With the shorter lengths of hospital stay and patients leaving the hospital in sicker and more debilitated states, this is particularly important to ensure there is adequate time to prepare the patient for discharge or to arrange for a post-discharge care setting. Astute discharge planning assists with giving a focus to outcomes, preventing complications, reducing the risk for readmission, and honoring the preferences of patients. Box 19.1 lists factors to consider in discharge planning. The need for specific types of assistance can be identified through a review of the factors on this list. It can be beneficial to provide a written list of medications and appointments, with related information, to ensure patients and their caregivers have the facts they need for future reference (see Boxes 19.2 and 19.3).

Box 19.1   Factors to Consider in Discharge Planning

- Patient's and caregivers' knowledge of the health condition and its care, and tests or studies that were completed and their outcomes
- Follow-up care required; scheduled appointments; patient's understanding of when and how to make appointments; ability to travel to appointments
- Patient and caregivers' understanding of steps to take if problems arise; their understanding of what would be considered an emergency situation that requires immediate attention and the actions to take
- Assistance the patient may need with activities of daily living and management of condition

(continued)

Box 19.1 *(Continued)*

- Caregivers' knowledge, skills, and comfort level in providing care, if applicable
- Medical equipment and supplies that will be needed; method for obtaining and paying for them; knowledge of proper use
- Patient's ability to obtain groceries and prepare meals
- Patient's and caregivers' understanding of medication purpose, administration times, routes, precautions, side effects, adverse effects to report; ability to obtain and pay for drugs
- Community resources that could assist patient and/or caregivers
- Other providers or agencies to whom discharge summary should be sent
- Preparation of written discharge plan and instructions

Box 19.2 Discharge Medication Record

Medication	Dose	When Taken	How to Take	Intended Purpose	Possible Side Effects	Effects to Report to Physician

Box 19.3   Appointment Schedule

Date	Name of Provider/ Lab/ Facility/ Agency	Location Address	Telephone Number	Preparation/ Points to Remember

In addition to considering the patient's needs in planning for discharge, thought must also be given to the family's needs and preferences. A patient may be resistant to be discharged to a nursing home and state that he or she can go home and be cared for by a daughter who lives in the same community. However, the daughter may have considerable responsibilities and not have the time or desire to provide daily care to her parent. If forced into this role, her own family and job may suffer and she may experience sufficient stress to cause health problems for herself. On the other hand, hospital staff may think that it is best for a patient to go to a nursing home because the patient's spouse, also of advanced age, is the only family member available to provide care. However, the spouse may prefer to care for his wife at home because he does not want to be separated from her, he derives a sense of purpose by caring for her, and he does not want to deplete their life savings for nursing home care. Realistic education, explanations, and counseling can aid families in making decisions that are effective and show concern for the patient and caregiver.

FAST FACTS in a NUTSHELL

The social services department of the hospital most likely will have a list of available home health agencies and nursing homes within the geographic area in which the patient lives that can assist with planning post-discharge care. In addition, the Centers for Medicare and Medicaid have a list of all home health agencies at www.medicare.gov/homehealthcompare and skilled nursing facilities at www.medicare.gov/nursinghomecompare. In addition to location and characteristics, the quality ratings of these home health agencies and nursing homes are provided on these sites.

NURSING HOMES

There are over 16,000 nursing homes in the United States, made up of a population largely over age 65 (Centers for Disease Control and Prevention, 2013b). Once a site in which people resided and received basic assistance with activities of daily living, nursing homes now are complex care centers. Growing numbers of people are admitted for short stays as they recover from major illnesses or receive rehabilitation, while there remains a population who will make the nursing home their home for the remainder of their lives.

FAST FACTS in a NUTSHELL

The complexities of today's nursing homes require nurses to be highly clinically competent in a wide range of specialties, as they may be caring for people who are receiving dialysis, cardiac rehabilitation, and ventilator support, as well as those with dementias and who have multiple chronic conditions that require management.

Nursing homes are monitored by government agencies that ensure the homes are meeting regulations. Federal regulations are the most minimum standards that nursing homes must meet (see Box 19.4); states can add to those regulations. The degree

Box 19.4 OBRA

In 1987 a major step in improving nursing home conditions was taken with the enactment of the Omnibus Budget Reconciliation Act of 1987, also known as the Nursing Home Reform Act of 1987 and commonly called OBRA. OBRA offered new minimum standards that aimed to improve care and grant nursing home residents' certain rights. Among the provisions are:

- A resident is to be assessed upon admission and at certain intervals thereafter using a uniform data form known as the Minimum Data Set (MDS) and have an individualized care plan developed based on assessment findings
- A resident's ability to perform activities of daily living should be maintained or improved unless there is a medical reason causing a decline
- Attention must be paid to preventing the development of pressure ulcers, unnecessary weight loss, dehydration, medication errors, and accidents
- Care must be provided to a resident who has urinary incontinence, and bladder function should be restored if possible
- Quality of life must be a concern in addition to quality of care; a resident must receive services that promote the quality of life to the fullest
- A resident has the right to be free from unnecessary or inappropriate physical and chemical restraints
- A resident has the right to return to the nursing home following a hospital stay or after an overnight visit with family or friends
- A resident has the right to remain in the nursing home unless there is a significant change in condition, the resident displays dangerous behaviors, or there is failure to pay for services
- A resident has the right to select a personal physician
- A resident has the right to access his or her medical records, and these records must be maintained accurately

(continued)

Box 19.4   (Continued)

- A resident has the right to form and participate in a resident or family council
- Family members cannot be forced to pay for services covered by Medicare and Medicaid
- A resident must be treated with dignity and respect

Surveyors evaluate the degree to which a nursing home meets OBRA standards through regular inspections. Nursing homes must meet these regulations in order to receive federal reimbursement for care. The Department of Health and Human Services (HHS) and state health departments may apply penalties against nursing homes for failure to meet the minimum standard of care as defined in the OBRA regulations. These penalties that a nursing home could face include fines, appointment of administrative consultants to run the nursing home while deficiencies are remedied, and closure.

A description of federal regulations and the survey process can be obtained at the Centers for Medicare and Medicaid Services website: www.cms.gov.

to which a nursing home meets these regulations is evaluated by surveys. Nursing homes must have satisfactory surveys to be licensed and certified. In addition to these basic standards, nursing homes can voluntarily choose to follow higher standards offered by The Joint Commission and develop their own set of additional standards. It is important for nurses employed in nursing homes to be familiar with the regulations and other standards they must follow.

One of the challenges for nurses who work in nursing homes is that nursing assistants deliver most direct care. Nurses often rely on these unlicensed workers to be the eyes and ears of changes in status, deliver care in a competent manner, and identify needs. Skillful guidance of these caregivers, good communication with them, and regular checks on their caregiving activities are crucial to ensure safe care.

=== *FAST FACTS in a NUTSHELL*

The American Association for Long Term Care Nursing offers several certification programs for nurses in various positions in nursing homes. Information can be obtained at www.ltcnursing.org.

Admission to a nursing home can be a highly stressful event for older individuals and their families. Many people have had minimal experience with nursing homes and hold negative views. Entering a nursing home often means major losses to older adults, such as status, roles, relationships, home, and finances. Family members may have a wide range of feelings about their loved one being admitted to a nursing home, ranging from guilt that they were unable to care for the person at home, to anger that they are faced with an added financial burden, to depression on seeing this change of condition and life circumstance of the person. Both the new resident and family members can be assisted during the admission process by:

- Greeting them as soon as they arrive, giving them a basic orientation to the facility, and ensuring they are comfortable (e.g., adequate chairs, offering drinks, informing them where bathrooms and vending machines are located).
- Describing resident and family rights and responsibilities.
- Writing down the names of the physician, director of nursing, administrator, unit charge nurse, direct care staff, social worker, and any other significant personnel; providing telephone contact numbers.
- Describing the anticipated sequence of events that will occur, as well as the typical day and routines (e.g., care plan conferences, activities, meal times, visiting hours).
- Encouraging them to ask questions.
- Being patient and understanding if communication and behaviors are less than positive. Remember that this is a highly stressful, emotionally filled time for them, and displacement of negative feelings to staff is not unusual.

Nursing homes that accept Medicare and Medicaid funding are required by the Centers for Medicare and Medicaid (CMS) to complete an admission tool for residents called the Minimum Data Set (MDS), which has sections pertaining to:

- Cognitive patterns
- Communication and hearing patterns
- Vision patterns
- Physical functioning and structural problems
- Continence
- Psychosocial well-being
- Mood and behavior patterns
- Activity pursuit patterns
- Disease diagnoses
- Other health conditions
- Oral/nutritional status
- Oral/dental status
- Skin condition
- Medication use
- Treatments and procedures

Nursing homes transmit their MDS tools electronically to the CMS and they enter this information into an MDS database for the respective states. The information provided in the tool determines the Resource Utilization Group (RUG) category, which ultimately determines the per diem rate paid to the facility for a resident whose stay is covered under Medicare Part A. This information is also part of the facility's quality indicator and quality measure reports, and can be examined by surveyors during nursing home inspections.

FAST FACTS in a NUTSHELL

The MDS tool must be completed on admission, annually, and whenever there is a change in the resident's condition.

The basic care of nursing home residents would be similar to patients in any setting with similar clinical diagnoses; however, there is another dimension to care that is unique in that the needs of people as *residents*, not just patients, of the facility must be considered. As many nursing home residents will remain in the facility for the remainder of their lives, creating a homelike environment becomes important. Related to this is attention to empowering and respecting the right of competent residents to make reasonable decisions related to their care, environment, and lives as though they were residing in their homes in the community.

FAST FACTS in a NUTSHELL

Culture change is a movement that began in the 1990s to create a more homelike environment in the nursing home and offer residents greater decision making, normalcy, and quality of life.

Many nursing homes have adopted culture change principles and practices, which include:

- Resident-centered care in which care activities are based on individual needs and preferences
- Holistic care that addresses needs of the body, mind, and spirit
- Consistency of staff assignments; empowerment of direct care staff
- Greater personalization of resident rooms
- Meals served more in restaurant or homelike fashion rather than on institutional-fashion trays; snacks available at all times
- Resident-directed care whereby residents determine schedules for bathing, eating, and other activities
- Environments that include attractive décor, plants, pets
- Creation of an inviting environment that promotes comfort and participation of visitors
- Provision of high-quality care

FAST FACTS in a NUTSHELL

The Pioneer Network is an organization that offers comprehensive information and many useful resources pertaining to culture change. Their website is www.PioneerNetwork.net.

ASSISTED LIVING COMMUNITIES

For people who need some assistance and supervision with care but do not have needs that would require the level and intensity of nursing home care, assisted living communities offer an option. These facilities tend to be more homelike than the typical nursing home and do not carry the stigma that has been associated with nursing homes, despite the reality that many assisted living communities care for people who are similar to nursing home residents. Some of these facilities offer specialized services, such as dementia care or hospice. Virtually all provide meals, assistance with medication administration, housekeeping and laundry services, and social programming. Trained staff are present, although there may not be a licensed nurse on at all times and in some models, a registered nurse only makes periodic visits to consult and is not present full time.

There is variation in physical plant, operations, size, and services provided among assisted living communities. Also, states vary in their regulatory requirements. Nurses are advised to check regulations pertaining to assisted living communities in their specific state and learn about the services, policies, staffing, and standards of individual communities in which they may be employed.

FAST FACTS in a NUTSHELL

A certification program for assisted living nurses is available from the American Assisted Living Nurses Association. Information can be obtained at www.alnursing.org.

HOME HEALTH

FAST FACTS in a NUTSHELL

In order for a patient's home care to be reimbursed by Medicare and some other insurance plans, it must be skilled. This means that the patient is homebound, care is required intermittently rather than full time, a primary care provider has ordered the services, and the services provided consist of skilled nursing or rehabilitation.

Home health agencies can provide anything from a short visit to change a dressing or check a patient's status to 24-hour nursing care, along with physical, occupational, and speech therapies. Although basic nursing care practices will be the same as nursing patients with similar conditions in any setting, some creativity and improvising may be necessary in the home settings. As most home health patients and their family caregivers will not have staff with them at all times, they need instruction as to potential risks and how to reduce them. This could include education about:

- Medications, their purpose, use, dosage, administration schedules, and adverse effects (writing this information on a form such as that shown in Box 19.2 is beneficial)
- Treatments and how to properly perform them
- Symptoms that are to be expected and those that might indicate a problem that should be promptly reported
- Transfer techniques
- Proper use of mobility aids and assistive devices

Home health nurses may need to anticipate potential problems such as those that could result from:

- The patient being unable to obtain groceries, prescriptions, or supplies due to lack of transportation or lack of funds
- The patient being too incapacitated to attend to paying rent, utilities, and other bills
- The home environment being dirty or infested with rodents or insects
- Safety risks in the home, such as scatter rugs, overloaded electrical outlets, broken door locks
- A pet that the patient has limited ability to care for or that has behaviors that could pose a risk
- The patient's isolation from neighbors or sources of help

When such problems are identified, the home health nurse needs to be proactive in assisting with finding a solution. Family members, social service agencies, and local faith communities can provide assistance that can make a significant difference in keeping the patient in his or her home.

OTHER GERIATRIC CARE SETTINGS

There are growing numbers of services tailored to meet the needs of older adults; in addition, there are many general health care programs that serve older adults along with other age groups. Among the settings for geriatric care are:

- *Adult day centers:* These centers offer social activities, medication management, assistance with personal care, monitoring of health conditions, and therapies. Usually the center transports the patient to and from the center where the patient spends approximately 8 hours.
- *Continuing care retirement communities:* Also known as life care centers, these communities offer a wide range of options for older adults that enable them to move along the health care continuum. Typically, the older person signs a contract with the community and lives in an independent style in an apartment or small house. As the patient needs care it can be provided within the person's home/apartment or, as needed, the person can move to other sections of the community that provide other levels of service. These settings offer a range of services for older adults, including health screening, health education, home visitation, home health care, primary care, adult day care, and nursing home care.
- *Health ministry services:* Many faith communities have nurses who are employed by or are volunteers in health ministry programs. These provide health screening, home visits, personal care assistance, and other health services.
- *Hospice:* Hospice programs provide care to persons at the end of life in the home or a facility dedicated to this purpose.
- *Respite care:* This service offers some relief for caregivers and can be effective for enabling dependent older adults to remain in the community rather than a nursing home. Respite care can consist of a health care worker staying in the home with the patient while the caregiver is away, a site where the patient can be taken to spend part of a day (such as an adult day center), or a short-term nursing home stay.
- *Subacute care:* Some hospitals and skilled nursing facilities operate units that have staffing, equipment, and resources to care for patients who do not require acute hospitalization

but who have complex, acute care needs that are beyond the capabilities of the average nursing home and/or that prevent them from being adequately cared for at home. Services could include ventilator care, complex wound care, chemotherapy, and intravenous therapy.

As can be seen, there is much diversity in geriatric care, which offers nurses many opportunities for challenging practice. As new models emerge, nurses play an important role in molding services to ensure older adults receive holistic, competent care.

Resources

Chapter 1

Bureau of Indian Affairs
www.doi.gov/bureau-indian-affairs.html

National Asian Pacific Center on Aging
www.napca.org

National Association for Hispanic Elderly
www.anppm.org

National Center on Black Aged
www.ncba-aged.org

National Center for Health Statistics
www.cdc.gov/nchs

National Hispanic Council on Aging
www.nhcoa.org

National Indian Council on Aging
www.nicoa.org

National Resource Center on Native American Aging
www.med.und.nodak.edu/depts/rural/nrcnaa/

Office of Minority Health Resource Center
www.omhrc.gov

Organization of Chinese Americans
www.ocanatl.org

SAGE (Services and Advocacy for Gay, Lesbian, Bisexual,
Transgender Elders)
www.sageusa.org/about/index.cfm

Chapter 2

Hartford Institute for Geriatric Nursing Try This Assessment Tool Series
hartfordign.org/practice/try_this/

Chapter 3

American Heart Association
www.heart.org

Mended Hearts (for patients with heart disease)
www.mendedhearts.org

National Heart, Lung, and Blood Institute
www.nhlbi.nih.gov

Chapter 4

American Lung Association
www.lungusa.org

Asthma and Allergy Foundation of America
www.aafa.org

National Heart, Lung, and Blood Institute Information Center
www.nhlbi.nih.gov

Office on Smoking and Health, Centers for Disease Control
and Prevention
www.cdc.gov/tobacco

Chapter 5

National Cancer Institute
www.cancer.gov

United Ostomy Association
www.uoa.org

Chapter 6

American Urologic Association
www.urologyhealth.org

Gilda's Club Worldwide
www.gildasclub.org

Gynecologic Cancer Foundation
www.wcn.org

MaleCare
www.malecare.com

National Association for Continence
www.nafc.org

National Breast Cancer Foundation
www.nationalbreastcancer.org

National Institute of Diabetes and Digestive and Kidney Diseases, National Kidney and Urologic Diseases Information Clearinghouse
www.kidney.niddk.nih.gov

National Prostate Cancer Coalition
www.fightprostatecancer.org

Ovarian Cancer National Alliance
www.ovariancancer.org

Simon Foundation for Continence
www.simonfoundation.org

Society of Urologic Nurses and Associates
www.suna.org

Chapter 7

Arthritis Foundation
www.arthritis.org

International Association of Yoga Therapists
www.iayt.org

National Arthritis and Musculoskeletal and Skin Diseases Information Clearinghouse
www.nih.gov/niams/

National Institute of Arthritis and Musculoskeletal and Skin Diseases (NIAMS)
www.niams.nih.gov

National Osteoporosis Foundation
www.nof.org

Chapter 8

Alexander Graham Bell Association for the Deaf
www.agbell.org

American Council of the Blind
www.acb.org

American Heart Association Stroke Connection
www.strokeassociation.org

American Humane Association Hearing Dog Program
www.americanhumane.org

American Parkinson Disease Association
www.apdaparkinson.org

American Speech-Language-Hearing Association
www.asha.org

Blinded Veterans Association
www.bva.org

Guide Dogs for the Blind
www.guidedogs.com

Guiding Eyes for the Blind
www.guiding-eyes.org

Leader Dogs for the Blind
www.leaderdog.org

Lighthouse National Center for Vision and Aging
www.lighthouse.org

Michael J. Fox Foundation for Parkinson's Research
www.michaeljfox.org

National Association for the Deaf
www.nad.org

National Library Service for the Blind and Physically Handicapped
www.lcweb.loc.gov/nls

National Institute of Neurological Disorders and Stroke
www.ninds.nih.gov

National Parkinson Foundation
www.parkinson.org

National Stroke Association
www.stroke.org

Paralyzed Veterans of America
www.pva.org

Parkinson Alliance
www.parkinsonalliance.org

Parkinson's Action Network (PAN)
www.parkinsonsaction.org

Parkinson's Disease Foundation (PDF)
www.pdf.org

Parkinson's Institute
www.thepi.org

Parkinson's Resource Organization
www.parkinsonsresource.org

Recordings for the Blind and Dyslexic
www.rfbd.org

Chapter 9

Agency for Healthcare Research and Quality
Pressure Ulcers in Hospitals: A Toolkit for Improving Quality of Care
www.ahrq.giv/researchltc/pressureulcertoolkit

American Academy of Facial and Reconstructive Plastic Surgery
www.aafprs.org/patient/procedures/proctypes.html

American Cancer Society
www.cancer.org

Braden Scale for Predicting Pressure Ulcer Risk
bradenscale.com/braden

National Arthritis and Musculoskeletal and Skin Diseases Information
Clearinghouse
www.nih.gov/niams

National Pressure Ulcer Advisory Panel
npuap.org

Skin Cancer Foundation
www.skincancer.org

Wound, Ostomy, and Continence Nursing Society
www.wocn.org

Chapter 10

American Diabetes Association
www.diabetes.org

American Heart Association
www.americanheart.org

National Diabetes Education Program
www.ndep.nih.gov

National Diabetes Information Clearinghouse
www.diabetes.niddk.nih.gov

Chapter 11

Al-Anon Family Group Headquarters (local chapters available)
www.al-anon-alateen.org

Alcoholics Anonymous (local chapters available)
www.alcoholics-anonymous.org

Alzheimer's Association
www.alz.org

Anxiety Disorders Association of America
www.adaa.org

Mental Health America
www.nmha.org

National Clearinghouse for Alcohol and Drug Information
www.ncadi.samhsa.gov/

National Depressive and Manic-Depressive Association
www.ndmda.org

National Institute of Alcohol Abuse and Alcoholism
www.niaaa.nih.gov

National Institute on Aging, Alzheimer's Disease Education
and Referral Center
www.nia.nih.gov/alzheimers

National Quality Forum Evidence Based Practices to
Treat Substance Abuse
www.qualityforum.org/projects/substance_use_2009.aspx

Chapter 12

BeliefNet
www.beliefnet.com

Duke Center for Spirituality, Theology, and Health
www.dukespiritualityandhealth.org

George Washington Institute for Spirituality and Health
www.gwish.org

Health Ministries Association
www.hmassoc.org

Nurses Christian Fellowship International
www.ncfi.org

Chapter 13

Arthritis Foundation
www.arthritis.org

Disabled American Veterans
www.dav.org

Dogs for the Deaf
www.dogsforthedeaf.org

Federal Government Disability Information
www.DisabilityInfo.gov

Guide Dogs for the Blind
www.guidedogs.com

Guiding Eyes for the Blind
www.guiding-eyes.org

Independent Living Aids
www.independentliving.com

Leader Dogs for the Blind
www.leaderdog.org

National Amputation Foundation
www.nationalamputation.org

National Braille Association
www.members.aol.com/nbaoffice

National Library Service for the Blind and Physically
Handicapped
www.loc.gov/nls

National Rehabilitation Information Center
www.naric.com

Paralyzed Veterans of America
www.pva.org

Sister Kenny Rehabilitation Institute
www.allina.com/ahs/ski.nsf

Chapter 14

AAA Foundation for Traffic Safety Senior Driver Website
www.seniordrivers.org/home/

Hartford Institute for Geriatric Nursing
Try This: Best Practices in Nursing Care to Older Adults Issue 8,
Fall Risk Assessment: Hendrich II Fall Risk Model
www.hartfordign.org/resources/education/ tryThis.html

National Center for Preparedness, Detection, and Control
of Infectious Diseases
www.cdc.gov/ncpdcid/

Chapter 15

Clearinghouse on Abuse and Neglect of the Elderly
www.elderabusecenter.org/clearing

Elder Mistreatment Assessment
consultgeri.org/resources

ElderWeb
www.elderweb.com

National Association of Professional Geriatric Care Managers
www.caremanager.org

National Center on Elder Abuse
www.ncea.aoa.gov

National Council on Family Relations
www.ncfr.com

National Eldercare Locator
www.eldercare.gov

National Family Caregivers Association
www.nfcacares.org

Chapter 16

American Geriatrics Society Beers List Guidelines and Clinical Tools
www.americangeriatrics.org/health_care_professionals/
clinical_practice/clinical_guidelines_recommendations/2012

Medications and You: A Guide for Older Adults
www.fda.gov/Drugs/ResourcesForYou/ucm163959.htm

Chapter 17

American Association of Retired Persons (AARP) Elder Law Forum
www.aarp.org/research/legal-advocacy/

American Bar Association Senior Lawyers Division
www.abanet.org/srlawyers/home.html

Hartford Institute for Geriatric Nursing
Try This: Best Practices in Nursing Care to Older Adults
Elder Mistreatment and Abuse Assessment
consultgerirn.org/topics/elder_mistreatment_and_abuse/
want_to_know_more

National Academy of Elder Law Attorneys
www.naela.com

National Center on Elder Abuse
www.elderabusecenter.org

National Senior Citizens Law Center
www.nsclc.org

Nursing Home Abuse/Elder Abuse Attorneys Referral Network
www.nursing-home-abuse-elderly-abuse-attorneys.com

Chapter 18

Advance Directives (by State)
www.noah-health.org/en/rights/endoflife/adforms.html
www.caringinfo/stateaddownload

American Hospice Foundation
www.americanhospice.org

End of Life/Palliative Education Resource Center
www.aacn.nche.edu/elnec/curriculum.htm

Family Hospice and Palliative Care
www.familyhospice.com

Hospice
www.hospicenet.org

Hospice Foundation of America
www.hospicefoundation.org

International Association for Hospice and Palliative Care
www.hospicecare.com

National Hospice and Palliative Care Organization
www.nhpco.org

Chapter 19

American Assisted Living Nurses Association
www.aalna.org

American Association of Nurse Assessment Coordination
www.aanac.org

American Association for Long-Term Care Nursing
www.LTCNursing.org

American Health Care Association
www.ahca.org

American Nurses Association, Inc., Council on Nursing Home Nurses
www.nursingworld.org

Eden Alternative
www.edenalt.org

Geriatric Advanced Practice Nursing Association
www.gapna.org

Green House Project
thegreenhouseproject.org

Leading Age (formerly American Association of Homes and Services for the Aging)
www.LeadingAge.org

National Association of Directors of Nursing Administration in Long-Term Care (NADONA)
www.NADONA.org

National Gerontological Nursing Association
www.ngna.org

Pioneer Network
www.pioneernetwork.net

The Consumer Voice for Quality Long Term Care
www.theconsumervoice.org

Recommended Readings

Chapter 1

Akincigil, A., Olfson, M., Siegel, M., Zurlo, K. A., Walkup, J. T., & Crystal, S. (2012). Racial and ethnic disparities in depression care in community-dwelling elderly in the United States. *American Journal of Public Health, 102*(2), 319–328.

Akushevich, I., Kravchenko, J., Ukraintseva, S., Arbeev, K., & Yashin, A. I. (2012). Age patters of incidence of geriatric disease in the U.S. population: Medicare-based analysis. *Journal of the American Geriatrics Society, 60*(2), 323–327.

American Association of Homes and Services for the Aging and Decision Strategies International. (2006). *The long and winding road. Histories of aging and aging services in America, 2006–2016.* Washington, DC: Author

American Journal of Nursing Continuing Education. (2006). *A new look at the old: A continuing education activity focused on healthcare for our aging population.* Philadelphia, PA: Lippincott Williams & Wilkins.

Andrews, M. M., & Boyle, J. S. (2008). *Transcultural concepts in nursing care* (5th ed.). Philadelphia, PA: Lippincott Williams & Wilkins.

Fredriksen-Goldsen, K. I., Kim, H.-J., Emlet, C. A., Muraco, A., Erosheva, E. A., Hoy-Ellis, C. P., … Petry, H. (2011). *The aging and health report: Disparities and resilience among lesbian, gay, bisexual, and transgender older adults.* Seattle, WA: Institute for Multigenerational Health.

Institute of Medicine. (2012). *The health of lesbian, gay, bisexual, and transgender people: Building a foundation for better understanding.* Washington, DC: National Academies Press. Available for free download at http://bit.ly/lRxMCf

National Center for Health Statistics. (2005). *Health, United States, 2005, with chartbook on trends in the health of Americans.* Hyattsville, MD: U.S. Department of Health and Human Services. Retrieved from http://www.cdc.gov/nchs/data/hus/hus05.pdf

Pruchno, R. (2012). Not your mother's old age: Baby boomers at age 65. *Gerontologist, 52*(2), 149–152.

Robinson, L. M., Dauenhauer, J., Bishop, K. M., & Baxter J. (2012). Growing health disparities for persons who are aging with intellectual and developmental disabilities. *Journal of Gerontology and Social Work, 55*(2), 175–190.

Sloan, F. A., Ayyagari, P., Salm, M., & Grossman, D. (2010). The longevity gap between black and white men in the United States at the beginning and end of the 20th century. *American Journal of Public Health, 100*(2), 357–363.

Villa, V. M., Wallace, S. P., Bagdasaryan, S., & Aranda, M. P. (2012). Hispanic baby boomers: Health inequities likely to persist in old age. *Gerontologist, 52*(2), 166–176.

Chapter 2

Boltz, M., Capezuti, E., Fulmer, T., & Zwicker, D. (2012). *Evidence-based geriatric nursing protocols for best practice* (4th ed.). New York, NY: Springer Publishing Company.

Clark, C. S. (2012). Beyond holism: Incorporating an integral approach to support caring-healing-sustainable nursing practices. *Holistic Nursing Practice, 26*(2), 92–102.

Corbett, C., Setter, S. M., Daratha, K. B., Neumiller, J. J., & Wood, L. D. (2010). Nurse identified hospital to home medication discrepancies: Implications for improving transitions of care. *Geriatric Nursing, 31*(3), 188–196.

Dickerson, J. B., Smith, M. L., Dowdy, D. M., McKinley, A., Ahn, S., & Ory, M. G. (2011). Advanced practice nurses' perspectives on the use of health optimization strategies for managing chronic disease among older adults in different care settings: Pushing the boundaries of self-management programs. *Geriatric Nursing, 32*(6), 429–438.

Digins, K. (2012). Hope yields health: Offering whole person care. *Journal of Christian Nursing, 29*(1), 11.

Jarvis, C. (2011). *Physical examination and health assessment* (6th ed.). St. Louis, MO: Saunders.

Koerner, J. G. (2011). *Healing presence: The essence of nursing* (2nd ed.). New York, NY: Springer Publishing Company.

Lindgren, C. L., & Murphy, A. M. (2002). Nurses' and family members' perceptions of nursing home residents' needs. *Journal of Gerontological Nursing, 28*(4), 45–53.

Mayo Clinic. (2006). *Mayo Clinic on healthy aging.* Rochester, MN: Author.

Steele, J. S. (2010). Current evidence regarding models of acute care for hospitalized geriatric patients. *Geriatric Nursing, 31*(5), 331–347.

Weinger, K. (2007). Psychosocial issues and self-care. *American Journal of Nursing, 107*(6, Suppl.), 34–38.

Chapter 3

Ancheta, I. B. (2006). A retrospective pilot study: Management of patients with heart failure. *Dimensions of Critical Care Nursing, 25*(5), 228–233.

Brown, T. J., & Mateko, E. B. (2005). Prevalence of hypertension in a sample of Black American adults using JNC 7 classifications. *Journal of the National Black Nurses Association, 16*(2), 1–5.

Corrigan, M. V., & Pallaki, M. (2009). General principles of hypertension management in the elderly. *Clinics in Geriatric Medicine, 25*, 207–212.

Handberg, E. (2006). End-of-life issues in elderly patients with acute coronary syndrome: The role of the cardiovascular nurse. *Progress in Cardiovascular Nursing, 21*(3), 151–155.

Mann, J. L., & Evans, T. S. (2006). A review of the management of heart failure in long-term care residents. *Consultant Pharmacist, 21*(3), 222–228.

Michael, K. M., & Shaughnessey, M. (2006). Stroke prevention and management in older adults. *Journal of Cardiovascular Nursing, 21*(5), S21–S26.

Ornish, D. (2008). *Dr. Dean Ornish's program for reversing heart disease.* New York, NY: Ivy Books.

Schipper, J. E., Coviellow, J., & Chyun, D. A. (2012). Fluid overload: Identifying and managing heart failure patients at risk for hospital readmission. In M. Boltz, E. Capezuti, T. Fulmer, & D. Zwicker(Eds.), *Evidence-based geriatric nursing protocols for best practice* (4th ed., pp. 628–657). New York, NY: Springer Publishing Company..

Chapter 4

Centers for Disease Control and Prevention. (2012). Lung cancer rates by race and ethnicity. Retrieved July 12, 2012, from http://www.cdc.gov/cancer/lung/statistics/race.htm

Cooley, M. E., Sipples, R. L., Murphy, M., & Sarna, L. (2008). Smoking cessation and lung cancer: Oncology nurses can make a difference. *Seminars in Oncology Nursing, 24*(1), 16–26.

Health Services Technology Assessment Text. (2008). Lung Cancer Screening: An Update for the U.S. Preventive Services Task Force, *U.S. Preventive Services Task Force Evidence Syntheses,* http://www.ncbi.nlm.nih.gov/books/bv. fcgi?rid=hstat3.section.33832.

Joyce, M., Schwartz, S., & Huhmann, M. (2008). Supportive care in lung cancer. *Seminars in Oncology Nursing, 24*(1), 57–67.

Lee, H., Kim, I., Lim, Y., Jung, H. Y., & Park, H. (2011). Depression and sleep disturbance in patients with chronic obstructive pulmonary disease. *Geriatric Nursing, 32*(6), 408–417.

Richards, C. L. (2007). Infection control in long-term care facilities. *Journal of the American Medical Directors Association, 8*(3, Suppl.), S18–S25.

Schweng, A. (2012). Flu shots. *American Journal of Nursing, 112*(2), 13.

Chapter 5

Burch, J. (2011). Management of stoma complications. *Nursing Times,* 107(45), 17–20.

Croft, L., & Prohlow, J. A. (2011). From fecal impaction to colon perforation. *American Journal of Nursing, 111*(8), 38–43.

Dahm, C. C., Keogh, R. H., Spencer, E. A., Greenwood, D. C., Ket, T. J., et al. (2010). Dietary fiber and colorectal cancer risk: A nested case-controlled study using food diaries. *Journal of the National Cancer Institute, 102*(9), 614–626.

Du, H., Van Der, A. D., Boshuizen, H. C., Forouhi, N. G., Wareham, N. J., et al. (2010). Dietary fiber and subsequent changes in body weight and waist circumference in European men and women. *Journal of Clinical Nutrition, 91*(2), 329–226.

Dyck, M. J., & Schumacher, J. R. (2011). Evidence-based practices for the prevention of weight loss in nursing home residents. *Journal of Gerontological Nursing, 37*(3), 22–33.

Franklin, L. E., Spain, M. P., & Edlund, B. J. (2012). Pharmacological management of chronic constipation in older adults. *Journal of Gerontological Nursing, 38*(4), 9–15.

Garcia, J. M., & Chambers, E. (2010). Managing dysphagia through diet modifications. *American Journal of Nursing, 110*(11), 26–33.

Ghezzi, E. M. (2012). Integration of oral health care into geriatric primary care: Proposal for collaboration. *Special Care Dentistry, 32*(3), 81–82.

Jablonski, R. A., Kolanowski, A. M., & Litaker, M. (2011). Profile of nursing home residents with dementia who require assistance with mouth care. *Geriatric Nursing, 32*(6), 439–446.

McHugh, M. E., & Miller-Saultz, D. (2011). Assessment and management of gastrointestinal symptoms of advanced illness. *Primary Care, 38*(2), 225–246.

Singh, M., & Tonk, R. S. (2012). Dietary considerations for patients with dry mouth. *General Dentistry, 60*(3), 188–189.

Chapter 6

Andriole, G. L., Crawford, E. D., Grubb, R. L. 3rd, Buys, S. S., Chia, D., Church, T. R., et al. (2012). PLCO Project Team. Prostate cancer screening in the randomized Prostate, Lung, Colorectal, and Ovarian Cancer Screening Trial: Mortality results after 13 years of follow-up. *Journal of National Cancer Institute, 104,* 125–132.

Aragon, D., & Sole, M. L. (2006). Implementing best practice strategies to prevent infection in the ICU. *Critical Care Nursing Clinics of North America, 18*(4), 441–452.

Baker, B., & Ward-Smith, P. (2012). Urinary incontinence nursing considerations at the end of life. *Urologic Nursing, 31*(3), 169–172.

Bernard, M. S., Hunter, K. F., & Moore, K. N. (2012). A review of strategies to decrease the duration of indwelling urethral catheters and potentially reduce the incidence of catheter-associated urinary tract infections. *Urologic Nursing, 32*(1), 29–37.

Breen, D. P., Wanserski, G. R., & Smith, P. C. (2007). Clinical inquiries. What is the recommended workup for a man with a first UTI? *Journal of Family Practice, 56*(8), 657–658, 661.

Bucci, A. T. (2007). Be a continence champion: Use the CHAMMP tool to individualize the plan of care. *Geriatric Nursing, 28*(2), 120–124.

Chou, R., Croswell, J. M., Dana, T., Bougatsos, C., Blazina, I., Fu, R., et al. (2011). Screening for prostate cancer: A review of the evidence for the U.S. Preventive Services Task Force. *Annals of Internal Medicine, 155*, 762–771.

Delancey, J. O. (2010). Why do women have stress urinary incontinence? *Neurourology and Urodynamics, 29*(Suppl. 1), 13–17.

Dowling-Castronovo, A. (2001). Urinary incontinence assessment. *Journal of Gerontological Nursing, 27*(5), 6–7.

Dowling-Castronovo, A., & Bradway, C. (2012). Urinary incontinence. *Evidence Based Geriatric Nursing Protocols for Best Practice* (pp. 363–387). New York, NY: Springer.

Dubeau, C. E. (2006). The aging lower urinary tract. *Journal of Urology, 175*(3), S11–S15.

Durrant, J., & Snape, J. (2003). Urinary incontinence in nursing homes for older people. *Age and Ageing, 32*(1), 12–18.

Gray, M. (2003). The importance of screening, assessing, and managing urinary incontinence in primary care. *Journal of the American Academy of Nursing Practice, 15*(3), 102–107.

Jackson, M. A. (2007). Evidence-based practice for evaluation and management of female urinary tract infection. *Urology Nursing, 27*(2), 133–136.

Jansen, L., & Forbes, B. (2006). The psychometric testing of a urinary incontinence nursing assessment instrument. *Journal of Wound, Ostomy, and Continence Nursing, 33*(1), 69–71.

Juthani-Mehta, M. (2007). Asymptomatic bacteriuria and urinary tract infection in older adults. *Clinics in Geriatric Medicine, 23*(3), 585–594.

LeCroy, C. (2006). Games as an innovative teaching strategy for overactive bladder and BPH. *Urology Nursing, 26*(5), 381–384, 393.

MacDonald, C. D., & Butler, L. (2007). Silent no more: Elderly women's stories of living with urinary incontinence in long-term care. *Journal of Gerontological Nursing, 33*(1), 14–20.

Matthews, P. A. (2007). Getting ready for certification: Bladder cancer. *Urology Nursing, 27*(3), 249–250.

McDougal, W. S., Wein, A. J., Kavoussi, L. R., & Novick, A. C. (2012). *Campbell-Walsh Urology* (10th ed.). Philadelphia, PA: Elsevier.

Miller, A. B. (2010). New data on prostate-cancer mortality after PSA screening [Editorial]. *New England Journal of Medicine, 366*, 1047–1048.

Moyer, V. A. (2012). Screening for Prostate Cancer: U.S. Preventive Services Task Force recommendations statement. *Annals of Internal Medicine, 156*(10), 812–825.

Nager, C. W., Brubaker, L., Litman, H. J., Zyczynski, H. M, Varner, R. E., et al. (2012). A randomized trial of urodynamic testing before stress-incontinence surgery. *New England Journal of Medicine, 366*(21), 1987–1997.

National Guideline Clearinghouse. (NGC). Guideline synthesis: Screening for prostate cancer. In: National Guideline Clearinghouse (NGC) [Web site]. Rockville (MD): Agency for Healthcare Research and Quality (AHRQ); 1998 Dec (revised 2013 Apr). Available at http://www.guideline.gov.

Newman, D. K. (2006). Urinary incontinence, catheters, and urinary tract infections: An overview of CMS tag F 315. *Ostomy and Wound Management, 52*(12), 34–36, 40–44.

Newman, D. K., & Koochaki, P. E. (2012). Characteristics and impact of interrupted sleep in women with overactive bladder. *Urologic Nursing, 31*(5), 304–312.

Palmer, H. H., & Newman, D. K. (2006). Bladder control educational needs of older adults. *Journal of Gerontological Nursing, 32*(1), 28–32.

Sanders, S., Bern-King, M., Specht, J., Mobily, P. R., & Bossen, A. (2012). Expanding the role of long-term care social workers: Assessment and intervention related to urinary incontinence. *Journal of Gerontological Social Work, 55*(3), 262–281.

Sublett, C. M. (2007). Adding to the evidence base—a critique of group session teaching of behavioral modification program for urinary incontinence. *Urology Nursing, 27*(2), 151–152.

Sublett, C. M. (2012). Adding to the evidence base: Efficacy of solifenacin for overactive bladder symptoms, symptom bother, and health-related quality of life in patients by duration of self-reported symptoms: A secondary analysis of the VIBRANT study. *Urologic Nursing, 32*(1), 47–49.

Wald, H. L., Fink, R. M., Makid, M. B. F., & Oman, K. S. (2012). Catheter-associated urinary tract infection prevention. *Evidence Based Geriatric Nursing Protocols for Best Practice* (pp. 388–408). New York, NY: Springer.

Williner, R., & Hantikainen, R. (2005). Individual quality of life following radical prostatectomy in men with prostate cancer. *Urology Nursing, 25*(2), 88–90.

Ziner, K. W., Sledge, G. W., Bell, C. J., Johns, S., Miller, K. D., & Champion, V. L. (2012). Predicting fear of breast cancer recurrence and self-efficacy in survivors by age at diagnosis. *Oncology Nursing Forum, 39*(3), 287–295.

Chapter 7

Anderson, J., White, K. G., & Kelechi, T. J. (2010). Managing common foot problems in older adults. *Journal of Gerontological Nursing, 36*(10), 9–14.

Egan, B. A., & Mentes, J. C. (2010). Benefits of physical activity for knee osteoarthritis: A brief review. *Journal of Gerontological Nursing, 36*(9), 9–14.

Fitzsimmons, S., & Schoenfelder, D. P. (2012). Evidence-based practice guideline: Wheelchair biking for the treatment of depression. *Journal of Gerontological Nursing, 37*(7), 8–15.

Greenblum, C. A., & Rowe, M. A. (2012). Nighttime activity in individuals with dementia: Understanding the problem and identifying solutions. *Journal of Gerontological Nursing, 38*(5), 8–11.

Jitramontree, N. (2010). Exercise promotion: Walking in elders. *Journal of Gerontological Nursing, 36*(11), 10–18.

Polzien, G. (2006). Care after hip replacement. *Home Healthcare Nurse, 24*(7), 420–422.

Schauff, J. (2011). Exploring the importance of OA and activity. *Journal of Gerontological Nursing, 37*(4), 5–6.

Williams, S. B., Brand, C. A., Hill, K. D., Hunt, S. B., & Moran, H. (2010). Feasibility and outcomes of a home-based exercise program on improving balance and gait stability in women with lower-limb osteoarthritis or rheumatoid arthritis: A pilot study. *Archives of Physical Medicine and Rehabilitation, 169*(21), 106–114.

Chapter 8

Amen, D. G. (2012). *Use your brain to change your age: Secrets to change your age.* New York, NY: Crown Publishing.

Bunting-Perry, L. K. (2006). Palliative care in Parkinson's disease: Implications for neuroscience nursing. *Journal of Neuroscience Nursing, 38*(2), 106–113.

Coombs, U. E. (2007). Spousal caregiving for stroke survivors. *Journal of Neuroscience Nursing, 39*(2), 112–119.

Fukunaga, A., Uematsu, H., & Sugimoto, K. (2005). Influences of aging on taste perception and oral somatic sensation. *Journal of Gerontology, Series A. Biological Sciences, 60*(1), 109–113.

Furie, K. L., Kasner, S. E., Adams, R. J., Albers, G. W., Bush, R. L., et al. (2012). Guidelines for the prevention of stroke in patients with stroke or transient ischemic attack: A guideline for healthcare professionals from the American Heart Association/American Stroke Association. *Stroke, 42*(1), 227–276.

Gupta, A., Epstein, J. B., & Sroussi, H. (2006). Hyposalivation in elderly patients. *Journal of the Canadian Dental Association, 72*(9), 841–846.

Habermann, B., & Davis, L. L. (2006). Lessons learned from a Parkinson's disease caregiver intervention pilot study. *Applied Nursing Research, 19*(4), 212–215.

Harper, J. P. (2007). Emergency nurses' knowledge of evidence-based ischemic stroke care: A pilot study. *Journal of Emergency Nursing, 33*(3), 202–207.

Hickey, J. V. (2012). *The Clinical Practice of Neurological and Neurosurgical Nursing.* Philadelphia, PA: Lippincott Williams & Wilkins.

Hinkle, J. (2005). An update on transient ischemic attacks. *Journal of Neuroscience Nursing, 37*(5), 243–248.

Kautz, D. D. (2007). Hope for love: Practical advice for intimacy and sex after stroke. *Rehabilitation Nursing, 32*(3), 95–103.

Lansbery, M. G., O'Donnell, M. J., Khatri, P., Lang, E. S., Ngugen-Huynh, M. N., et al. (2012). Antithrombotic and thrombolytic therapy for ischemic stroke: Antithrombotic Therapy and Prevention of Thrombosis (9th ed.): American College of Chest Physicians Evidence-Based Clinical Practice Guidelines. *Chest, 141*(2, Suppl.), 601–636.

Mathiesen, C., Tavianini, H. D., & Palladino, K. (2006). Best practices in stroke rapid response: A case study. *MedSurg Nursing, 15*(6), 364–369.

Ney, D., Weiss, J., Kind, A., & Robinson, J. A. (2009). Senescent swallowing: Impact, strategies and interventions. *Nutrition in Clinical Practice, 24*(3), 395–413.

Phillips, L. J. (2006). Dropping the bomb: The experience of being diagnosed with Parkinson's disease. *Geriatric Nursing, 27*(6), 362–369.

Rabbitt, P., Scott, M., Lunn, M., Thacker, N., Lowe, C., et al. (2007). White matter lesions account for all age-related declines in speed but not in intelligence. *Neuropsychology, 21*(3), 363–370.

Snyder, C. H., & Adler, C. H. (2007). The patient with Parkinson's disease: Part I-Treating the motor symptoms; Part II-Treating the nonmotor symptoms. *Journal of the American Academy of Nurse Practitioners, 19*(4), 179–197.

Thomure, A. (2006). Helping your patient manage Parkinson's disease. *Nursing 2006, 36*(8), 20–21.

Vacca, V. M. (2007). Acute paraplegia. *Nursing 2007, 37*(6), 64.

Wysong, A., Lee, P. P., & Sloan, F. A. (2010). Longitudinal incidence of adverse outcomes of age-related macular degeneration. *Archives of Ophthalmology, 127,* 320–327.

Chapter 9

Ayello, E. A., & Sibbald, R. G. (2012). Preventing pressure ulcers and skin tears. In *Evidence-based geriatric nursing protocols for best practice* (pp.298–323). New York, NY: Springer Publishing Company.

Black, J., Baharestani, M., Cuddigan, J., Dormer, B., Edsberg, L., et al. (2007). National Pressure Ulcer Advisory Panel's updated pressure ulcer staging system. *Dermatology Nursing, 19*(4), 343–349.

Bolton, L. (2010). Pressure ulcers. In J. M. MacDonald & M. J. Geyer (Eds.), *Wound and lymphedema management* (pp. 95–101). Geneva, Switzerland: World Health Organization.

Burt, T. (2013). Palliative care of pressure ulcers in long term care. *Annals of Long-Term Care, 21*(3), 20–28.

Campbell, K. E., Woodbury, M. G., & Houghton, P. E. (2010). Implementation of best practice in the prevention of heel pressure ulcers in the acute orthopedic populations. *International Wound Journal, 7*(1), 28–40.

Cho, I., & Noh, M. (2010). Braden Scale: Evaluation of clinical usefulness in an intensive care unit. *Journal of Advanced Nursing, 66*(2), 293–302.

Consortium for Spinal Cord Medicine. (2007). Pressure ulcer prevention and treatment following spinal cord injury: A clinical practice guideline for health care professionals. Guideline available at http://www.pva.org . Washington, DC: Paralyzed Veterans of America.

Iezzoni, L. I., & Ogg, M. (2012). Hard lessons from a long hospital stay . *American Journal of Nursing, 112*(4), 39–42.

Langemo, D. (2012). General principles and approaches to wound prevention and care at end of life: An overview?. *Ostomy and Wound Management, 58*(5), 24–34.

Scalf, L. A., & Shenefeld, P. D. (2007). Contact dermatitis: Diagnosing and treating skin conditions in the elderly. *Geriatrics, 62*(6), 14–19.

Stafiej, J. M., & Szewczyk, M. T. (2012). Treatment of full-thickness pressure ulcers with a gentamicin sponge: A case report. *Journal of Wound, Ostomy, and Continence Nursing, 39*(3), 331–341.

Tosta de Souza, D. M. S., Conceica de Santos, V. L., Keiko, H., & Oquiri, M. Y. S. (2010). Predictive validity of the Braden Scale for pressure ulcer risk in elderly residents of long term care facilities. *Geriatric Nursing,31*(2), 95–104.

Chapter 10

American Diabetes Association. (2007). Standards of medical care in diabetes—2007. *Diabetes Care, 30*, S4–S41.

Astle, F. (2007). Diabetes and depression: A review of the literature. *Nursing Clinics of North America, 42*(1), 67–78.

Bass, A., Will, T., Todd, M., & Weatherford, D. (2007). The latest tools for patients with diabetes. *RN 2007, 70*(6), 39–43.

Behr, M. (2007). Diabetes. *Medical Surgical Nursing, 16*(2), 122–123.

Bolen, S., Feldman, L., Vassy, J., Wilson, L., Yeh, H. C., et al. (2007). Systematic review: Comparative effectiveness and safety of oral medications for type 2 diabetes mellitus. *Annals of Internal Medicine, 147*(6), 178–180.

Burton, J. E. (2011). Hyperthyroidism. *Medsurg Nursing, 20*(3),152–153.

Funnell, M. M. (2012). Understanding insulin resistance. *Nursing, 42*(3),62.

Funnell, M. M., Brown, T. L., Childs, B. P., Haas, L. B., Hosey, G. M., et al. (2007). National standards for diabetes self-management education. *Diabetes Care, 30*(6), 1630–1637.

Gore, T. N., Williams, A., & Sanderson, B. (2012). Recipe for health: Impacting diabetes in African Americans through faith-based education. *Journal of Christian Nursing, 29*(1),49–53.

Grant, R. W., Wexler, D. J., Ashburner, J. M., Hong, C. S., & Atlas, S. J. (2012). Characteristics of "complex" patients with type 2 diabetes mellitus according to their primary care physicians. *Archives of Internal Medicine*, 28(10), 821–823.

Grontved, A., & Hu, F. B. (2011). Television viewing and risk of type 2 diabetes, cardiovascular disease, and all-cause mortality. A meta-analysis. *Journal of the American Medical Association*, 305(23), 2248–2255.

Harris, C. (2007). Recognizing thyroid storm in the neurologically impaired patient. *Journal of Neuroscience Nursing*, 39(1), 40–42, 57.

Kapustin, J. F. (2010). Hypothyroidism: An evidence-based approach to a complex disorder. *Nurse Practitioner*, 35(8), 44–53.

Miller, J. (2007). Diabetes and thyroid disease: Nursing care to improve outcomes for patients living in poverty. *Nursing Clinics of North America*, 42(1), 113–125.

Monami, M., Luzzi, C., Lamana, C., Chiaserrini, V., Adante, F., et al. (2007). Three-year mortality in diabetic patients treated with different combinations of insulin secretagogues and metformin. *Diabetes/Metabolism Research Review*, 22(6), 477–482.

Munt, R., & Hutton, A. (2012). Type 1 diabetes mellitus (T1DM) self management in hospital; is it possible? A literature review. *Contemporary Nurse*, 40(2), 179–193.

Nissen, S. E. (2012). Cardiovascular effects of diabetes drugs: Emerging from the dark ages. *Annals of Internal Medicine*, 157(9), 671–672.

Oxtoby, K. (2012). Improving diabetes care. *Nursing Times*, 108(10), 27.

Roumie, C. L., Hung, A. M., Greevy, R. A., Grijalva, C. G., Liu, X., et al. (2012). Comparative effectiveness of sulfonylurea and metformin monotherapy on cardiovascular events in type 2 diabetes mellitus: A cohort study. *Annals of Internal Medicine*, 157(9), 601–610.

Salem, J. K., Jones, R. R., Sweet, D. B., Hasan, S., Torregosa-Arcay, H. & Clough, L. (2011). Improving care in a resident practice for patients with diabetes. *Journal of Graduate Medical Education*, 3(2), 196–202.

Seley, J. A., & Weinger, K. (2007). Executive summary. The state of the science on nursing best practices for diabetes self-management. *American Journal of Nursing*, 107 (6, Suppl.), 6–11.

Simmons, S. (2010). A delicate balance: Detecting thyroid disease. *Nursing*, 40(7):22–29.

Wang, R. H., Lin, L. Y., Cheng, C. P., Hsu, M. T., & Kao, C. C. (2012). The psychometric testing of the diabetes health promotion self-care scale. *Journal of Nursing Research*, 20(2), 122–130.

Whittemore, R. (2006). Behavioral interventions for diabetes self-management. *Nursing Clinics of North America*, 41(4), 641–654.

Whittemore, R. (2007). Culturally competent interventions for Hispanic adults with type 2 diabetes. *Journal of Transcultural Nursing*, 18(2), 15–66.

Yen, P. (2002). Treating diabetes with diet. *Geriatric Nursing*, 23(5), 175–176.

Zarowitz, B. (2006). Management of diabetes mellitus in older persons. *Geriatric Nursing, 27*(1), 77–82.

Chapter 11

Adelman D. S., Legg T. J. (2010). Caring for older adults with dementia when disaster strikes. *Journal of Gerentological Nursing, 36*(8), 13–17.

Amen, D. G. (2012). *Use your brain to change your age: Secrets to change your age.* New York: Crown Publishing.

Beck, C., Buckwater, K. C., Dudzik, P. M., & Evans, L. K. (2011). Filling the void in geriatric mental health: The Geropsychiatric Nursing Collaborative as a model for change. *Nursing Outlook, 59*(4), 236–241.

Clarke, S. P., McRae, M. E., Del Signore, S., Schubert, M., & Styra, R. (2010). Delirium in older cardiac surgery patients: Directions for practice. *Journal of Gerontological Nursing, 36*(11), 34–45.

DiBartolo, M. C. (2012). Dementia revisited. *Journal of Gerontological Nursing, 38*(5), 46–51.

Flanagan, N. M. (2011). Driving and dementia: What nurses need to know. *Journal of Gerontological Nursing, 37*(8), 10–13.

Gage, S., & Melillo, K. D. (2011). Substance abuse in older adults: Policy issues. *Journal of Gerontological Nursing, 37*(12), 8–11.

Gerdner, L. A., & Schoenfelder, D. P. (2010). Evidence-based guideline. Individualized music for elders with dementia. *Journal of Gerontological Nursing, 36*(6), 7–15.

Gould, R. L., Coulson, M. C., & Howard, R. J. (2012). Efficacy of cognitive behavioral therapy for anxiety disorders in older people: A meta-analysis and meta-regression of randomized controlled trials. *Journal of the American Geriatrics Society, 60*(2), 218–229.

Green, L., Matos, P., Murillo, I., Neushotz, L., Popeo, D., et al. (2011). Use of dolls as a therapeutic intervention: Relationship to previous negative behaviors and pro re nata (prn) Haldol use among geropsychiatric inpatients. *Archives of Psychiatric Nursing, 25*(5), 388–389.

Greenberg, S. A. (2007). How to try this: The Geriatric Depression Scale: Short Form. *American Journal of Nursing, 107*(10), 60–69.

Hahn, J. E. (2012). Minimizing health risks among older adults with intellectual and/or developmental disabilities: clinical considerations to promote quality of life. *Journal of Gerontological Nursing, 38*(6), 11–17.

Holliday-Welsh, D. M., Gessert, C. E., & Renier, C. M. (2009). Massage in the management of agitation in nursing home residents with cognitive impairment. *Geriatric Nursing, 30*(2), 109–117.

Kolanowski, A. (2011). An invitation to a conversation on quality of life in dementia. *Journal of Gerontological Nursing, 37*(2), 4–5.

Lane, A. M. & Hirst, S. P. (2012). Are gerontological nurses apathetic about apathy in older adults. *Journal of Gerontological Nursing, 38*(1), 22–28.

Legg, T. J., & Adelman, D. S. (2011). Diagnosis: Dementia. Psychiatric referral versus federal regulations: a balancing act for long-term care nurses. *Journal of Gerontological Nursing, 37*(11), 24–27.

Lu, D. F., & Herr, K. (2012). Pain in dementia: Recognition and treatment. *Journal of Gerontological Nursing, 28*(2), 8–13.

Naegle, M. (2012). Substance misuse and alcohol use disorders. In M. Boltz, E. Capezuti, T. Fulmer, & D. Zwicker (Eds.), *Evidence-based geriatric nursing protocols for best practice* (pp. 516–543). New York, NY: Springer Publishing Company.

Paun, O., & Farran, C. J. (2011). Chronic grief management for dementia caregivers in transition: Intervention development and implementation. *Journal of Gerontological Nursing, 37*(12), 28–35.

Rose, K. M., & Williams, I. C. (2011). Family matters. Family quality of life in Dementia. *Journal of Gerontological Nursing, 37*(6), 3–4.

Schultz, S. K. (2011). The hazardous territory of late-life depression: A challenge to geropsychiatry. *American Journal of Geriatric Psychiatry, 19*(3), 197–200.

Slaughter, S. E., Morgan, D., & Drummond, N. (2011). Functional transitions of nursing home residents with middle-stage dementia. *Journal of Gerontological Nursing, 37*(5), 50–59.

Specht, J. T., (2011). Promoting continence in individuals with dementia. *Journal of Gerontological Nursing, 37*(2), 17–21.

Steis, M. R., & Fick, D. M. (2012). Delirium superimposed on dementia: Accuracy of nurse documentation. *Journal of Gerontological Nursing, 38*(1), 32–42.

Vance, D. E., Eagerton, G., Harnish, B., McKie, P, & Fazeli, P. L. (2011). Cognitive prescriptions. *Journal of Gerontological Nursing, 37*(4), 22–29.

Wierman, H. R., Wadland, W. R., Walters, M., Kuhn, C., & Farrington, S. (2011). Nonpharmacological management of agitation in hospitalized patients. *Journal of Gerontological Nursing, 37*(2), 44–48.

Chapter 12

Anderson, M., & Burggraf, V. (2007). Passing the torch: Transcendence. *Geriatric Nursing, 28*(1), 37–38.

Autry, J. A. (2002). *The spirit of retirement. Creating a life of meaning and personal growth.* New York: Prima Press.

Barnum, B. S. (2006). *Spirituality in nursing* (2nd ed.). New York, NY: Springer Publishing Company.

Callen, B. L., Mefford, L., Groer, M., & Thomas, S. P. (2011). Relationships among stress, infectious illness, and religiousness/spirituality in community-dwelling older adults. *Research in Gerontological Nursing, 4*(3), 195–206.

Houston, J. M., & Parker, M. (2011). *A vision for the aging church: Renewing ministry for and by seniors.* Downers Grove, IL: Intervarsity Press.

Kellemen, R. W., & Edwards, K. A. (2007). *Beyond suffering: Embracing the legacy of African American soul care and spiritual direction*. Grand Rapids, MI: Baker Books.

King, M.A., & Pappas-Roqich, M. (2011). Faith community nurses: Implementing healthy people standards to promote the health of elderly clients. *Geriatric Nursing, 32*(6): 459–464.

Koenig, H. G. (2011). *Spirituality and Health Research*. New York, NY: Templeton Press.

Sun, F., Park, N. S., Roff, L. L., Klemmack, D. L., Parker, M., Koenig, H. G., … Allman, R. M. (2012). Predicting the trajectories of depressive symptoms among southern community-dwelling older adults: The role of religiosity. *Aging and Mental Health, 16*(2), 189–198.

Wang, J. J. (2012). A structural model of the bio-psycho-socio-spiritual factors influencing the development towards gerotranscendence in a sample of institutionalized elders. *Journal of Advanced Nursing, 67*(12), 2628–2636.

Chapter 13

Couzner, L., Radcliffe, J., & Crotty, M. (2012). The relationship between quality of life, health and care transition: An empirical study of an older post-acute population. *Health and Quality of Life Outcomes, 10*(1), 69.

Donesky, D. A., Janson, S. L., Nguyen, H. Q., Neuhaus, J., Neilands, T. B., & Carrier-Kohlman, V. (2011). Determinants of frequency, duration, and continuity of home walking in patients with COPD. *Journal of Gerontological Nursing, 32*(3), 178–187.

Eliopoulos, C. (2010). Deconditioning and Sarcopenia. *Long-Term Living, 59*(3), 14–15.

Enguidanos, S., Gibbs, N., & Jamison, P. (2012). From hospital to home: A brief nurse practitioner intervention for vulnerable older adults. *Journal of Gerontological Nursing, 38*(3), 40–50.

Fagard, R. H. (2012). Physical activity, fitness, and mortality. *Journal of Hypertension, 30*(7), 1310–1312.

Park, J., & McCaffrey, R. (2012). Chair yoga: Benefits for community dwelling older adults with osteoarthritis. *Journal of Gerontological Nursing, 38*(5), 12–25.

Chapter 14

Centers for Disease Control and Prevention. (2007). Falls in nursing homes. National Center for Injury Prevention and Control, Centers for Disease Control and Prevention. Retrieved from http://www.cdc.gov/ncipc/factsheets/ nursing.htm

Cheung, S. S. (2007). Neuropsychological determinants of exercise tolerance in the heat. *Progressive Brain Research, 165*, 45–60.

Gray-Miceli, D., & Quigley, P. A. (2012). Fall prevention: Assessment, diagnoses, and intervention strategies. In M. Boltz, E. Capezuti, T. Fulmer, D. & Zwicker (Eds.), *Evidence-based geriatric nursing protocols for best practice* (4th ed.). New York, NY: Springer Publishing Company.

Gray-Miceli, D., Ratcliff, S. J., & Johnson, J. C. (2010). Use of a postfall assessment tool to prevent falls. *Western Journal of Nursing Research, 32*(7), 932–948.

Ko, A., Nguyen, H. V., Chan, L., Shen, Q., Ding, A. M., et al. (2012). Developing a self-reported tool on fall risk based on toileting responses on in-hospital falls. *Geriatric Nursing 33*(1), 9–16.

Palmisano-Mills, C. (2007). Common problems in hospitalized older adults. *Journal of Gerontological Nursing, 33*(1), 48–54.

Quigley, P., & Goff, L. (2011). Current and emerging innovations to keep patients safe. Technological innovations play a leading role in fall-prevention programs. Special Report: Best Practices for Fall Reduction. A practice guide. *American Nurse Today,* March, 14–17.

Shields, W. C., Perry, E. C., Szanton, S. L., Andrews, M. R., Stepnitz, E. M., et al. (2013). Knowledge and injury prevention practices in homes of older adults. *Geriatric Nursing, 34*(1):19–24.

Voukelatos, A., Cumming, R. G., Lord, S. R., & Rissel, C. (2007). A randomized, controlled trial of tai chi for the prevention of falls: The central Sydney tai chi trial. *Journal of the American Geriatrics Society, 55*(8), 1185–1191.

Wiens, C. A., Coleba, T., Jones, C. A., & Feeney, D. F. (2006). The Falls Risk Awareness Questionnaire: Development and validation for use with older adults. *Journal of Gerontological Nursing, 32*(8), 43–50.

Chapter 15

Acierno, R., Hernadez, M. A., Amstadter, A. B., Resnick, H. S., Steve, K., et al. (2010). Prevalence and correlates of emotional, physical, sexual, and financial abuse and potential neglect in the United States: The National Elder Mistreatment Study. *American Journal of Public Health, 100*(2), 292–297.

Boltz, M. (2012). The family caregiver: An untapped resource. *Geriatric Nursing, 33*(2), 137–139.

Caceres, B., & Fulmer, T. (2012). Mistreatment detection. In M. Boltz, E. Capezuti, T. Fulmer, & D. Zwicker (Eds.), *Evidence-based geriatric nursing practice* (4th ed., pp. 544–561). New York, NY: Springer.

Chang, H. Y., Chiou, C. J., & Chen, N. S. (2010). Impact of mental health and caregiver burden on family caregivers' physical health. *Archives of Gerontology and Geriatrics, 50*(2), 267–271.

Cohen, C. J., Auslander, G., & Chen, Y. (2010). Family caregiving to hospitalized end-of-life and acutely ill geriatric patients. *Journal of Gerontological Nursing, 36*(8), 42–50.

Hirst, S. P. (2012). Grandparenting today is changing gerontological nursing practice. *Journal of Gerontological Nursing, 38*(4), 3–4.

Hoffman, G .J., Lee, J., & Mendez-Luck, C. A. (2012). Health behaviors among Baby Boomer informal caregivers. *Gerontologist, 52*(2), 219–230.

Kagan, S. H. (2011). Resident and family-centered care. Is there individualized care here? *Geriatric Nursing, 32*(5), 365–367.

Mast, M. E., Sawin, E. M., & Pantaleo, K. A. (2012). Life of a caregiver simulation: Teaching students about frail older adults and their family caregivers. *Journal of Nursing Education, 51*(4), 1–7.

Palmer, J. L. (2012). Caregivers' desired patterns of communication with nursing home staff—just TALKK. *Journal of Gerontological Nursing, 38*(4), 47–54.

Pruchno, R. (2012). Not your mother's old age: Baby boomers at age 65. *Gerontologist, 52*(2), 149–145.

Ume, E. P., & Evans, B. C. (2011). Chaos and uncertainty: The post-caregiving transition. *Geriatric Nursing, 32*(4), 288–293.

Wiglesworth, A., Mosqueda, L., Mulnard, R., Liao, S., Gibbs, L., & Fitzgerald, W. (2010). Screening for abuse and neglect of people with dementia. *Journal of the American Geriatrics Society, 58*(3), 493–500.

Chapter 16

American Geriatrics Society 2012 Beers Criteria Update Expert Panel. (2012). The American geriatrics society updated beers criteria for potentially inappropriate medication use in older adults. *Journal of the American Geriatrics Society, 60*(4), 616–631.

Bergman-Evans, B. (2006). AIDES to improving medication adherence in older adults. *Geriatric Nursing, 27*(3), 174–175.

Bergman-Evans, B. (2006). Evidence-based guideline. Improving medication management for older adult clients. *Journal of Gerontological Nursing, 32*(7), 6–14.

Fick, D. M., & Resnick, B. (2012). 2012 Beers Criteria update: How should practicing nurses use the criteria? *Journal of Gerontological Nursing, 38*(6), 3–5.

Hoskins, B. L. (2011). Safe prescribing for the elderly. *Nurse Practitioner, 36*(12), 47–52.

Howland, R. H. (2011). Update on newer antipsychotic drugs. *Journal of Psychosocial Nursing and Mental Health Services, 49*(4), 13–15.

Martin, D., Kripalani, S., & DuRapau, V. J. (2012). Improving medication management among at-risk older adults. *Journal of Gerontological Nursing, 38*(6), 36–37.

Mitsch, A. L. (2013). Antidepressant adverse drug reactions in older adults: Implications for RNs and APNs. *Geriatric Nursing, 34*(1), 53–60.

Monroe, T., Carter, M., & Parish, A. (2011). A case study using the beers list criteria to compare prescribing by family practitioners and geriatric specialists in a rural nursing home. *Geriatric Nursing, 32*(5), 350–356.

Patterson, S. M., Hughes, C., Kerse, N., Cardwell, C. R., & Bradley, M. C. (2012). Interventions to improve the appropriate use of polypharmacy for older people. *Cochrane Database System Review, 16*(5), CD008165.

Peron, E. P., Gray, S. L., & Hanlon, J. T. (2011). Medication use and functional status decline in older adults: A narrative review. *American Journal of Geriatric Pharmacotherapy, 9*(6), 378–391.

Ruppar, T. M., Dobbels, F., & DeGeest, S. (2012). Medication beliefs and antihypertensive adherence among older adults: A pilot study. *Geriatric Nursing, 33*(2), 89–95.

Stuart, R. L., Wilson, J., Bellaard-Smith, E., Brown, R., Wright, L., Vandergraaf, S., & Gillespie, E. E. (2012). Antibiotic use and misuse in residential aged care facilities. *Internal Medicine Journal, 4*, 1445–1459.

Wehling, M. (2012). *Drug therapy for the elderly.* New York, NY: Springer Publishing Company.

Zarowitz, B. J. (2013). Comprehensive medication review: Coming soon to a nursing home near you! *Geriatric Nursing, 34*(1), 62–65.

Chapter 17

Adelman, R. (2013). Assisted living lawsuits: An ounce of prevention is worth a pound of cure. *Geriatric Nursing, 34*(2):166–169.

Allen, J. (2011). Resident care decisions in assisted living: Who is in charge? *Geriatric Nursing, 24*(1), 146–147.

American Bar Association. (2007). Factbook on the law and the elderly, http://www.abanet.org/media/factbooks/ eldtoc.html

Grant, P. D., & Ballard, D. (2011). Law for nurse leaders: A comprehensive approach. New York, NY: Springer.

Guido, G. W. (2009). Legal and ethical issues in nursing (5th ed.). New York, NY: Prentice Hall.

Kapp, M. B. (2010). Legal aspects of elder care. Sudbury, MA: Jones & Bartlett.

Lynch, V. A., & Duval, J. B. (2010). Forensic nursing science (2nd ed.). St Louis, MO: Elsevier.

Mitty, E. L., & Post, L. F. (2012). Health care decision making. In M. Boltz, E. Capezuti, T. Fulmer, & D. Zwicker (Eds.), *Evidence-based geriatric nursing protocols for best practice*, (4th ed., pp. 562–578). New York, NY: Springer.

Wiglesworth, A., Mosqueda, L., Liao, S., Gibbs, L., & Fitzgerald, W. (2010). Screening for abuse and neglect of people with dementia. *Journal of the American Geriatrics Society, 58*, 493–500.

Chapter 18

Allen, J. (2010). The POLST: Advocating for assisted living residents' end-of-life wishes. *Geriatric Nursing, 31*(3), 234–235.

Choi, M., Lee, J., Kim, S., Kim, D., & Kim, H. (2012). Nurses' knowledge about end-of-life care: Where are we? *Journal of Gerontological Nursing,42*(6), 61–65.

Cohen, C. J., Auslander, G., & Chen, Y. (2010). Family caregiving to hospitalized end-of-life and acutely ill geriatric patients. *Journal of Gerontological Nursing, 36*(8), 42–50.

Dorfman, J., Denduluri, S., Walseman, K., & Bregman, B. (2012). The role of complementary and alternative medicine in end-of-life care. *Psychiatric Annals, 42*(4), 150–155.

Gordon, M. (2013). Care demands by families and family healthcare proxies: A dilemma for palliative care and hospice staff. *Annals of Long Term Care 21*(5), 42–46.

Hansen, L., Cartwright, J. C., & Craig, C. E. (2012). End-of-life care for rural-dwelling older adults and their primary family caregivers. *Journal of Gerontological Nursing, 5*(1), 6–15.

Hartford Geriatric Nursing Initiative. (2013). *Try this: Assessing pain in older adults.* John A. Hartford Foundation for Geriatric Nursing, http://hartfordign.org/Resources/Try_This_Series.

Maltoni, M., Scarpi, E., & Rosati, M. (2012). Palliative sedation in end-of-life care and survival: A systematic review. *Journal of Clinical Oncology, 30*(12), 1378–1383.

McCabe, M. P., Mellor, D., Davison, T. E., Hallford, D. J., & Goldhammer, D. L. (2012). Detecting and managing depressed patients: Palliative care nurses' self-efficacy and perceived barriers to care. *Journal of Palliative Medicine, 15*(4), 463–467.

Mitty, E. (2012). Advance directives. In M. Boltz, E. Capezuti, T. Fulmer, & D. Zwicker(Eds.), *Evidence-based geriatric nursing protocols for best practice* (4th ed., pp. 579–599). New York, NY: Springer.

Remington, R., & Wakim, G. (2010). A comparison of hospice in the United States and the United Kingdom: Implications for practice. *Journal of Gerontological Nursing,36*(9), 16–21.

Senft, D. J. (2011). Home health and hospice face-to-face encounter visits. *Geriatric Nursing,32*(6), 450–452.

Tuck, I., Johnson, S. C., Kuznetsova, M. I., McCrockli, C., Baxter, M., & Bennington, L. K. (2012). Sacred healing stories told at the end of life. *Journal of Holistic Nursing, 30*(2), 69–80.

Chapter 19

Balas, M. C., Casey, C. M., & Happ, M. B. (2012). Comprehensive assessment and management of the critically ill. In M. Boltz, E. Capezuti,

T. Fulmer, & D. Zwicker (Eds.), *Evidence-based geriatric nursing protocols for best practice* (4th ed., pp. 600–627). New York, NY: Springer Publishing Company.

Bobay, K. L., Jerofke, T. A., Weiss, M. E., & Yakusheva, O. (2010). Age-related differences in perception of discharge planning teaching and readiness for hospital discharge. *Geriatric Nursing, 31*(3), 178-187.

Bradas, C. M., Sandhu, S. K., & Mion, L. C. (2012). Physical restraints and side rails in acute and critical care settings. In M. Boltz, E. Capezuti, T. Fulmer, & D. Zwicker (Eds.), *Evidence-based geriatric nursing protocols for best practice* (4th ed., pp. 229–245). New York, NY: Springer Publishing Company.

Cherry, B. (2011). Assessing organizational readiness for electronic health record adoption in long-term care facilities. *Journal of Gerontological Nursing, 37*(10), 14–19.

Eliopoulos, C. (2012). *Nursing administration of long-term care facilities* (8th ed.). Glen Arm, MD: Health Education Network.

Eliopoulos, C. (2013). *Culture change nurse coordinator manual* (3rd ed.). Glen Arm, MD: Health Education Network.

Enguidanos, S., Gibbs, N., & Jamison, P. (2012). From hospital to home: A brief nurse practitioner intervention for vulnerable adults. *Journal of Gerontological Nursing, 38*(3), 40–50.

Ferrari, M., Harrison, B., Rawashdeh, O., Hammond, R., Avery, Y., et al. (2012). *Geriatric Nursing, 33*(3), 177–183.

Francis, D. C., & Lahaie, J. M. (2012). Iatrogensis: The nurse's role in preventing patient harm. In M. Boltz, E. Capezuti, T. Fulmer, D. & Zwicker (Eds.), *Evidence-based geriatric nursing protocols for best practice* (4th ed., pp. 200-228). New York, NY: Springer Publishing Company.

Houde, S. C., Melillo, K. D., & Holmes, R. (2012). The patient-centered medical home. *Journal of Gerontological Nursing, 38*(3), 12–16.

Huckstadt, A. A. (2002). The experience of hospitalized elderly patients. *Journal of Gerontological Nursing, 28*(9), 24–29.

Ko, A., Nguyen, H. V., Chan, L., Shen, Q., Ding, A. M., et al. (2012). Developing a self-reported tool on fall risk based on toileting responses on in-hospital falls. *Geriatric Nursing, 33*(1), 9–16.

Markley, J., Andow, V., Sabharwal, K., Wang, Z., Fennell, E., & Dusek, R. (2013). A project to reengineer discharges reduces 30-day readmission rates. *American Journal of Nursing, 113*(7), 55–64.

May, K. N., & Mion, L. C. (2013). Nurses' impact on the hospital environment: Lessening or contributing to the chaos? *Geriatric Nursing 34*(1), 72–74.

Mueller, C., Burger, S, Rader, J., & Carter, D. (2013). Nurse competencies for person-directed care in nursing homes. *Geriatric Nursing, 34*(2), 101–104.

Palmer, J. L. (2012). Caregivers' desired patterns of communication with nursing home staff—just TALKK. *Journal of Gerontological Nursing, 38*(4), 47–54.

Rantz, M. J., Skubic, M., Koopman, R. J., Alexander, G. L., Phillips, L., et al. (2012). Automated technology to speed recognition of signs of illness in older adults. *Journal of Gerontological Nursing, 38*(4), 18–23.

Steele, J. S. (2010). Current evidence regarding models of acute care for hospitalized geriatric patients. *Geriatric Nursing, 31*(5), 331–347.

Stefanacci, R. G. (2013). Care coordination today: What, why, who, where, and how? *Annals of Long Term Care, 21*(3), 38–42.

Steis, M. R., & Fick, D. M. (2012). Delirium superimposed on dementia: Accuracy of nurse documentation. *Journal of Gerontological Nursing, 38*(1), 32–42.

Tsai, H. H., & Tsai, Y. F. (2011). Changes in depressive symptoms, social support, and loneliness over one year after a minimum three month videoconference program for older nursing home residents. *Journal of Medical Internet Research, 13*(4), 93–95.

Wang, C., Fetzer, S. J., Yang, Y., & Wang, J. (2013). The impact of using community health volunteers to coach medication safety behaviors among rural elders with chronic illnesses. *Geriatric Nursing, 34*(2), 138–145.

Wu, M. L., Courtney, M. D., Shortridge-Baggett, L. M., Finlayson, K., & Isenring, E. A. (2012). Validity of the malnutrition screening tool for older adults at high risk of hospital readmission. *Journal of Gerontological Nursing, 38*(6), 38–45.

References

Administration on Aging. (2012). *Minority aging.* Retrieved April 10, 2012, from http://www.aoa.gov/AoARoot/Aging_Statistics/Minority_Aging/index.aspx

Alzheimer's Association. (2013). Alzheimer's disease facts and figures. *Alzheimer's & Dementia, 9*(2), 15.

American Cancer Society. (2007). *Detailed guide: Breast cancer. What are the risk factors for breast cancer? Retrieved from* http://www.cancer.org/docroot/CRI/content/CRI_2_4_2X_What_are_the_risk_factors_for_breast_cancer_5.asp

American Cancer Society. (2012). *What are the key statistics for bladder cancer? Cancer reference information.* Retrieved January 16, 2013, from http://www.cancer.org/cancer/bladdercancer/detailedguide/bladder-cancer-key-statistics

American College of Obstetricians and Gynecologists. (2013). *Routine screening recommendations released for annual well woman exam.* Retrieved February 2, 2013, from http://www.acog.org

American Diabetes Association. (2010). Executive summary: Standards of medical care of diabetes 2010. *Diabetes Care, 33*(S1), S4–S10.

American Psychiatric Association. (2013). *Diagnostic and statistical manual of mental disorders* (5th ed.). Washington, DC: Author.

Bates-Jensen, B. M. (1996). Why and how to assess pressure ulcers. Presented at the Ninth Annual Symposium on Advanced Wound Care, Atlanta, April 20, 1996.

Bergstrom, M., Allman, R. M., & Carlson, E. D. (1994). Treatment of pressure ulcers. Clinical Practice Guideline No. 15, AHCPR Pub No 95-0652. Rockville, MD: U.S. Department of Health and Human Services, Public Health Service, Agency for Health Care Policy and Research.

Blanchard-Fields, F., & Kalinauskas, A. (2009). Theoretical perspectives on social context, cognition, and aging. In V. L. Bengston, M. Silverstein, N. M. Putney, & D. Gans (Eds.), *Handbook of theories of aging* (2nd ed., pp. 261–276). New York: Springer.

Centers for Disease Control and Prevention, Data and Statistics. (2011). Retrieved May 10, 2013, from http://www.cdc.gov/injury/wisqars/fatal.html

Centers for Disease Control and Prevention, National Center for Injury Prevention and Control, Division of Unintentional Injury Prevention. (2012). *Costs of falls among older adults.* Retrieved May 10, 2013, from http://www.cdc.gov/HomeandRecreationalSafety/Falls/fallcost.html

Centers for Disease Control and Prevention. (2013). *Black women have higher rates of death from breast cancer than other women.* Retrieved January 11, 2013, from http://www.cdc.gov/vitalsigns/BreastCancer/index.html

Centers for Disease control and Prevention. (2013). *Falls among older adults: An overview.* Retrieved March 5, 2013, from http://www.cdc.gov/HomeandRecreationalSafety/Falls/adultfalls.html

Centers for Disease Control and Prevention. (2013). *Diabetes Fact Sheet 2011.* Available at http://www.cdc.gov/diabetes/pubs/pdf/ndfs_2011.pdf

Centers for Disease Control and Prevention. (2013a). *Hospital utilization.* Retrieved July 9, 2013, from http://www.cdc.gov/nchs/fastats/hospital.htm

Centers for Disease Control and Prevention. (2013b). Fast facts, nursing home care. Retrieved June 19, 2013, from http://www.cdc.gov/nchs/fastats/nursingh.htm

Chen, L. H., Warner, M., Fingerhut, L., & Makuc, D. (2009). Injury episodes and circumstances: National Health Interview Survey, 1997–2007. National Center for Health Statistics. *Vital Health Statistics, 10*(241), 14.

Dasgupta, M., & Hillier, L. M. (2010). Factors associated with prolonged delirium: A systematic review. *International Psychogeriatrics, 22*(3), 373–394.

Fredriksen-Goldsen, K. I., Kim, H.-J., Emlet, C. A., Muraco, A., Erosheva, E. A., Hoy-Ellis, C. P., … Petry, H. (2011). *The aging and health report: Disparities and resilience among lesbian, gay, bisexual, and transgender older adults.* Seattle, WA: Institute for Multigenerational Health.

Harvath, T. A. & McKenzie, G. (2012). Depression in older adults. In M. Boltz, E. Capezuti, T. Fulmer, & D. Zwicker (Eds.) *Evidence-based geriatric nursing protocols for best practice* (pp. 141–142). New York: Springer Publishing Company.

Horn, E. P., Bein, B., Bohm, R., Steinfath, M., Sahili, N., & Hocker, J. (2012). The effect of short time periods of pre-operative warming in the prevention of peri-operative hypothermia. *Aneasthesia, 67*(6), 612–617.

Jones, E. T., Stephenson, K. W., King, J. G., Knight, K. R., Marshall, T. L., & Scott, W. B. (2009). Sarcopenia: Mechanisms and treatments. *Journal of Geriatric Physical Therapy*, 32(2), 83–89.

Jurgens, C. Y., Hoke, L., Byrnes, J., & Riegel, B. (2009). Why do elders delay responding to heart failure symptoms? *Nursing Research*, 58(4), 274–282.

Keller, M. (2011). Dealing with dysphagia. *Aging Well*, 4(1), 8.

Kübler-Ross, E. (1969). *On death and dying*. New York, NY: Macmillan.

Lapid, M. I., Prom, M. C., Burton, M. C., McAlpine, D. E., Sutor, B., & Rummans, T. A. (2010). Eating disorders in the elderly. *International Journal of Psychogeriatrics*, 22(4), 523–536.

Lerma, E. V. (2009). Anatomic and physiologic changes of the aging kidney. *Clinics in Geriatric Medicine*. 25, 325–329.

McKhann, G. M., Knopman, D. S., Chertkow, H., Hyman, B. T., Jack, C. R., Kawas, C. H., ... Phelps, C. H. (2011). The diagnosis of dementia due to Alzheimer's disease: Recommendations from the National Institute on Aging-Alzhemier's Association workgroups on diagnostic guidelines for Alzheimer's disease. *Alzheimer's & Dementia*, 7(3), 263–269.

National Cancer Institute. (2013). Observation as good as surgery for some men with prostate cancer. Retrieved January 15, 2013 from http://www.cancer.gov/clinicaltrials/results/summary/2012/prostate-observation0912

National Center for Elder Abuse. (2013). Fact sheet about elder abuse. Retrieved June 2, 2013, from http://www.ncea.aoa.gov/Resources/Publication/docs/FinalStatistics050331.pdf

National Institute of Neurological Disorders & Stroke, National Institutes of Health. (2013). Neuroleptic Malignant Syndrome (NMS). Retrieved May, 2013, from http://www ninds.nih.gov/disorders/neuroleptic.syndrome/

National Institutes of Health. (2004). The Seventh Report of the Joint National Committee on Prevention, Detection, Evaluation, and Treatment of High Blood Pressure, page 30. Retrieved November 3, 2012, from http://www.nhlbi.nih.gov/guidelines/hypertension/jnc7full.pdf

Norton, D., McLaren, R., & Exton-Smith, A. N. (1962). *An investigation of geriatric nursing problems in the hospital*. London: National Corporation for the Care of Old People.

Pickering, T. G., Miller, N. H., Ogedebe, G., Krakoff, L. R., Artinana, N. T., & Goff, D. (2008). Call to action on use and reimbursement for home blood pressure monitoring. *Journal of Cardiovascular Nursing*, 23, 299–323.

Poggio, R., Grancelli, H. O., & Miruka, S. G. (2010). Understanding the risk of hyperkalemia in heart failure: Role of aldosterone antagonism. *Postgraduate Medical Journal*, 86(1013), 136–142.

Ridker, P. M. (2003). Clinical application of C-reactive protein for cardiovascular disease detection and prevention. *Circulation*, 107(3), 363–369.

Sampson, N., Untergasser, G., Plas, E., & Berger, P. (2007). The aging male reproductive tract. *Journal of Pathology, 211*(2), 206–218.

Shallenbarger, S. (2012). Safer over 70: Drivers keep the keys. Wall Street Journal, February 29, 2012, page D3.

Steinman & Hanlon. (2010). Managing medications in clinically complex elder: There's got to be a happy medium. *Journal of the American Medical Association, 304*(14), 1592–1601.

Strachan, M. W., Reynolds, R. M., Marioni, R. E., & Price, J. F. (2011). Cognitive function, dementia and type 2 diabetes mellitus in the elderly. *National Review of Endocrinology, 7*(2), 108–114.

U.S. Census Bureau. (2012). Figure 11, Percent distribution of population age 65 and over by race and Hispanic oridi: 1990 to 2050. *Population projections of the United States by age, sex, race, and Hispanic origin: 1995 to 2050*. Retrieved December 19, 2012, from http://www.census.gov/prod/1/pop/p25-1130.pdf

U.S. Food and Drug Administration. (2005). FDA public health advisory: Deaths from antipsychotics in elderly patients with behavioral disturbances. Retrieved August 10, 2007, from http://www.fda.gov/Cder/drug/advisory/ antipsychotics.htm

VanGilder, C., Amlung, S., Harrison, P., & Meyer, S. (2009). Results of the 2008-2009 International Pressure Ulcer Prevalence Survey and a 3-year, acute care, unit-specific analysis. *Ostomy/Wound Management, 55*(11), 39-45.

Watson, L. C., Zinnerman, S., Cohen, L. W., & Dominik, R. (2009). Practical depression screening in residential care assisted living: Five methods compared with gold standard diagnoses. *American Journal of Geriatric Psychiatry, 17*(7), 556–564.

Wilson, R. S., Hebert, L. E., Scherr, P. A., Dong, X., Leurgens, S. E., & Evans, D. A. (2012). Cognitive decline after hospitalization in a community population of older persons. *Neurology, 78*(3), 950–956.

Yang, H. L., Lee, H. F., Chu, T. L., Su, Y. Y., Ho, L. L., & Fan, J. Y. (2012). The comparison of two recovery room warming methods for hypothermia patients who had undergone spinal surgery. *Journal of Nursing Scholarship, 44*(1), 2–10.

Index